Living Life Well

New Strategies for Hard Times

Living Life Well

New Strategies for Hard Times

Patricia Robinson, Ph.D.

CONTEXT PRESS
Reno, Nevada

Living Life Well: New Strategies for Hard Times, by Patricia Robinson

Paperback. 111 pp. Includes bibliographies.

Distributed by New Harbinger Publications, Inc.

Living life well : new strategies for hard times / by Patricia Robinson
p. cm.
ISBN-13: 978-1-878978-27-1 (pbk.)
ISBN-10: 1-878978-27-6 (pbk.)

1996 CONTEXT PRESS
933 Gear Street, Reno, NV 89503-2729

Dedicated to

people

who see opportunities

in their suffering

Acknowledgments

Until just now, I thought acknowledgment meant expression of appreciation. To stimulate my listing of people I appreciate, I looked up the meaning of acknowledgment and found that it was closer to "find a middle course" than to "thank you." Larger efforts in our lives evolve from and through interactions with many people. Some are joyful and some are painful and some just are. These are the people who struggled with me and helped me write down the compromises suggested in this book: Kirk Strosahl, Wanda Johnson, Merl E. Bonney, E. Robert Sinnett, James Coyne, Virginia Jolly, Karen Hagen, and Taj Worley. Others helped me "shape it up," including Scott Compton, Judith Lull Strosahl, Carrie Utic, Connie Schnell, and Christi Landrum-Ricchi. My three daughters made helpful concessions with me during my writing time. Thank you--Regan, Frances, and Joanna--for helping me "strike a balance." Finally, I acknowledge the many patients who invested their trust and confidence in me.

Table of Contents

Living Life Well: New Strategies for Hard Times

Introduction

Depression is very common today. Anxiety and stress reactions are also prevalent. This book is a self-management workbook. Use it! Write in it! It can help you learn from difficult experiences and recover from a personal crisis with more skills and greater confidence. Troubled relationships can improve. Your productivity at work can return. You do not need to "get stuck" in patterns of suffering that continue for years.

This book will help you to recognize the parts of your life that work well and **attend more closely** to those areas that are working *less well*. I will suggest strategies and exercises to help you create more satisfying experiences in life on a day-to-day basis. As a starting point, slow down and reflect for a moment. If you look back over your last ten years, you probably recall some good times and some not-so-good. Focus for a moment on a time in your life during the past few years when you were contented. What was happening then? What made your life satisfying? What was your daily routine? Where did you work? Who were your friends? This kind of "creative daydreaming" may help you find "clues" for making changes in your present life. This book will present you with many opportunities to exercise your imagination for the benefit of your life.

What makes life worthwhile for you? For most of us, life is good when we find meaning or purpose in our daily activities. Even during the most stressful times, we know contentment when we choose to "live our values." Here's another exercise for you to consider. Take a few minutes to sit outside and breathe in fresh air. If you prefer to sit inside, sit in your favorite chair, relax, and ask yourself, "What is most important in life?" Listen for answers. Listen for your own personal truth about the "meaning of life" for you. These are the guides to consult when you plan your day. Use the following format to help you clarify what is most important to you in seven basic areas of living.

In The Following 7 Contexts Of Life, My Guiding Values Are:	
Life Context	**Value**
Personal Growth or Development	
Leisure Activities	
Family Relationships	
Marriage or Intimate Relationship	
Work	
Community Involvement	
Spiritual Experience	

Harry Stack Sullivan once said, "We are all more alike than different." While your values may differ from your friends or loved ones in small ways, they are probably quite similar in many ways. We value security and the ability to make choices about our leisure activities and our spiritual practices. We want to find meaning in our work. We admire kindness, thoughtfulness, intelligence, courage, and health. We want to feel mentally and physically "well."

Numerous psychology and health care researchers are investigating psychological and biological components of well-being. Recently, Dr. Michael Dougher suggested that well-being is present when the following qualities distinguish your day-to day life.

- You "live" your values.

- You are open to your thoughts, images, and feelings.

- You interact with friends.

- Your actions are truthful.

- You accept yourself, and you accept others.

- You feel vital.

- You are productive in the work you choose to do.

How many of these characteristics were on your list of values? Keep your list of values. Add to it as you make discoveries. Perhaps you can make your list into a book marker to use in reading the rest of this book.

Keeping reminders of your values nearby is a good idea because they are easy to forget when you are overwhelmed. My grandmother had 13 different artistic displays of the serenity prayer in her four-room house. She was a nurse and she lived through the "Great Depression." She lost two husbands and worked mostly with dying patients. I wondered about all those serenity prayers as a child. Now, I understand that they gave meaning to suffering. The verse reminded her to accept her daily experiences of loss and sadness *and still make room* for the joy of being in her garden, reading the comics, and playing with her pets.

Whether the challenges you face today are new or long-standing, you can use this book to gain a better understanding of your response to them. I encourage you to take the time to evaluate your coping efforts on a weekly basis for the next month or two. **Commit to practicing suggested exercises.** Experimentation, practice, and perseverance will help you "live well"--even during "hard times."

Over the past 20 years, I have learned a lot from my patients. I have learned a great deal about coping with adversity. The strategies I present in this book have worked for many people. In fact, **most of the ideas in this book were evaluated in a large scientific study**. In this study, we found that people who made a sustained effort to practice suggested exercises and apply recommended strategies experienced the following rewards.

1. More enjoyment of daily activities

2. More effective coping on a daily basis

3. More skillful problem-solving

4. Greater optimism about the future

5. More tranquillity and satisfaction

6. Improved sense of physical and psychological well-being

This study took place in a health care center. Some of the people in the study had health problems. Others struggled with financial hardships. Almost half reported job problems. A clear majority felt very sad about problems in their closest relationships. We compared two groups. One group received care only from their health care team. The other group used materials from this book and support from a behavioral health professional working with their health care team. The second group was much more improved than the first at follow-ups one, four and seven months later.

Support from others is very important when you try to change your behavior. In the study, the people who benefited from working with materials similar to this book received three to five hours of support from health care professionals over a six-month period. Some of you may be able to provide your own support. Others will need support from a friend or professional. Who will support you for taking the time needed to read this book and implement plans to improve the quality of your life? Your helper can be a friend or loved one. Alternatively, your supporter could be your primary care nurse, physician, or a behavioral health specialist. Make a note concerning who will provide support to you.

The person who is most able to help me is:

If you are suffering a great deal at this point, consider contacting a mental health professional. This book is not a substitute for psychotherapy. Appendix A presents information to help you select a counselor or psychologist. Many mental health professionals will be willing to help you work through the seven-week program suggested in this book. If you see a mental health professional and plan to use this program in treatment, suggest that she or he read the companion book for mental health professionals, titled *Treating Depression in Primary Care: A Manual for Primary Care and Mental Health Providers.* You are far more likely to complete this book and benefit from it if you have one or more people in your life pulling for you. Identify your helper(s) now.

Sometimes, medications are an important part of recovery from the debilitating physiological effects of acute or on-going stressful circumstances. Medications can be used in combination with the behavioral and acceptance strategies suggested in this book. Additional information concerning use of medications is presented in Appendix B. If you are interested in using medication, complete the form in Appendix C. Plan a visit to your primary care physician. Take your responses to questions in Appendix C with you when you go to discuss medication treatment with your physician. If you start antidepressant treatment, become familiar with the strategies about using medications that are presented in Appendix D. Use the form below to indicate your plan regarding medication.

Yes	No	**Your Decision Concerning Medications**
		I am not interested in medication at present.
		I am interested in medications.
		I plan to complete the form in Appendix C and visit my physician.

I will present two general approaches to coping in this book. The first approach may be more familiar to you than the second. The first focuses on behavior and lifestyle changes. In Chapter 1, you will learn the basics of behavioral change. You will apply behavioral change strategies to develop *behavioral health plans* as you progress through the remaining chapters. In Chapter 2, I present a second approach to coping – psychological acceptance. Acceptance strategies offer a powerful alternative to behavioral change strategies for some problems (Hayes & Strosahl, 1996). For other problems, psychological acceptance strategies complement and strengthen behavioral change plans. Throughout the book, I will suggest ways of combining behavioral change and acceptance strategies.

In Chapter 3, I suggest several methods for working with your body. Recent research results indicate that mental events are also physical events. All thoughts have a biological parallel. Dr. Deepak Chopra advises us to "stop looking at the human body as a body and a mind, or as a mind inside a body, and view it instead as a body/mind" (Chopra, 1994, p. 10). Chapter 3 is intended to help you work with your *body/mind*.

In Chapter 4, you will learn a set of guidelines to use to solve current problems in your life. In 1995, Drs. Mynors-Wallace and Gath reported that people who worked with their family physicians to apply skills similar to those in Chapter 4 benefited greatly. In fact, they experienced as much improvement in mood as people who used antidepressant medications.

Chapters 5 and 6 present acceptance and behavioral change strategies to help you improve your relationships with others and express yourself in creative activities. Conflict with loved ones is one of the most common causes of discouragement and depression. Successful resolution of conflict requires personal commitment and interpersonal skillfulness. Well-established patterns of effective assertion and creative expression can provide a substantial buffer to stress.

In the last chapter, I suggest a method to help you maintain gains you make from applying strategies suggested in this workbook. While you are likely to feel much better a month from now, you will still be vulnerable to future stresses and associated depression and anxiety. Your newer patterns of behavior will lack the strength that comes with longer-term practice. The last chapter helps you develop an effective plan for *continuing* to live life well.

There are seven chapters in this book. Every chapter has seven sections. The "Chapter Sections" table summarizes the structure within each chapter. **You do not need to read the entire book to benefit** from the program suggested. If you are unsure of the relevance of a particular chapter to your life, skim the second section of the chapter (i.e., "Strategies") to get a quick description of strategies included in that chapter.

Table: Chapter Sections	
Chapter Sections	**Purpose of Section**
1. Self-Assessment	Helps you develop change plans and evaluate your progress.
2. Strategies	Provides an overview of coping strategies presented in the chapter.
3. Effectiveness	Provides a synopsis of relevant research findings concerning the effectiveness of the strategies presented.
4. Goal Setting	Assists you with setting a goal concerning use of suggested strategies.
5. Skill Work	Presents exercises to help you clarify potential uses of suggested strategies in your life.
6. Example	Illustrates how you can apply suggested strategies to improve quality of life.
7. Behavioral Health Plan	Provides a format for developing a written behavioral health change plan.

In using this book, you can follow one of two programs. The "Options" table summarizes the two programs. Reading and completing exercises in Chapters 1, 2, 3, 4, and 7 constitute the basic, bare-bones life improvement program. This program is called the "Basic Program." In the "Enhanced Program," you enrich the Basic Program by including Chapters 5 and 6 in your plan. Chapters 5 presents methods for working with yourself and with others when there is conflict. Chapter 6 suggests strategies for assertively and creatively expressing yourself on a day-to-day basis.

The ideas in Chapters 5 and 6 will help you become more resilient to the negative impact of stress in the future. They are well worth your time.

In all chapters you choose to read, take time to **complete the suggested written activities**. Some chapters may be more relevant to you than others. When you reach a chapter that is particularly meaningful for your life, slow your pace and practice more. Work at a regular pace. Most people will be able to complete a chapter in 3 to 7 days. I recommend that you plan to use one or more activities suggested in this book on a *daily* basis for the next two months. This type of commitment will maximize your chances of long-term benefit. While some of the exercises may be fun, others may be difficult and painful. **Decide now to stay with the program. Living life well requires intention and persistence**.

Table: Options		
Program	**Chapter**	**Objective**
Basic Program		**Chapters 1, 2, 3, 4, and 7**
	1	Increasing Hopefulness and Skills for Making Behavioral Health Plans
	2	Increasing Psychological Acceptance Skills and Ability to Make Value-Based Plans
	3	Increasing Skills for Creating Sensations of Wellness
	4	Increasing Skills for Problem-Solving
	7	Planning a Lifestyle that Reflects Your Values
Enhanced Program		**Chapters 1, 2, 3, 4, and 7 plus 5 and 6**
	5	Increasing Skills for Responding to Interpersonal Conflict
	6	Increasing Skills for Assertive and Creative Expression
I plan to use this book to complete the:		☐ 1. The Basic Program
		☐ 2. The Enhanced Program

After you complete this book and graduate to a new level in living your life well, I suggest that you keep the book around for a while. When life comes at you "hard and fast" again, skim this book. Review your responses to questions and exercises in the book. *Remember* what helped you most during your first reading of the book. Start the acceptance and change process *again*.

References

Chopra, D. (1994). *Restful Sleep: The complete mind/body program for overcoming insomnia*. New York, NY: Harmony Books.

Hayes, S. C., Strosahl, K. D., & Wilson, K. G. (1999*). Acceptance and commitment therapy: An experiential approach to behavior change*. New York, NY: Guilford Press.

Katon, W., Robinson, P., Von Korff, M., Lin, E., Bush, T., Ludman, E., Simon, G., & Walker, E. (1996). A multifaceted intervention to improve treatment of depression in primary care. *Archives of General Psychiatry, 53*(10), 924-932.

Mynors-Wallace, L., Gath, D. H., Lloyd-Thomas, A. R., & Tomlinson, D. (1995). Randomized controlled trial comparing problem-solving treatment with amitriptyline and placebo for major depression in primary care. *British Medical Journal, 310*, 441-446.

Robinson, P., Bush, T., Von Korff, M., Katon, W., Simon, G., Walker, E., & Lin, E. (1996). Educational materials for depressed primary care patients and subsequent use of suggested coping strategies. Submitted for Publication.

Robinson, P., Katon, W., Von Korff, M., Bush, T., Ludman, E., Simon, G., Lin, E., & Walker, E. (1996). Use of coping strategies by depressed primary care patients: Results of a randomized controlled trial. In preparation for submission.

Chapter 1

Hoping . . . Planning . . . Doing

In this chapter, you will have an opportunity to select a method for keeping track of how you are doing. Also, you will critically examine your *explanation* of current difficulties. Your interpretation of a challenging circumstance can be a source of depression *or* inspiration. In this chapter, you learn to "fertilize" your own sense of hopefulness by working with your thoughts.

Additionally, I present the basics of the behavioral change strategy in this chapter. You will have your first chance to make a behavioral health plan to improve the quality of your life. You will apply these behavioral change skills to one of seven areas of your life on a weekly basis as you progress through this book. These skills are critically important to effective self-management.

This may sound like a lot of work right now. Keep reading. Exercises in this chapter will help you develop hope. With a little hope, your energy for experimenting and learning will grow. Let's start with several methods for increasing awareness of your day-to-day experience in life.

Self-Assessment

On-going self-assessment helps you become more aware of the quality of your life on a daily basis. Further, monitoring helps you evaluate the impact of using new strategies and allows you to see your progress over time. There are three approaches to self-assessment designed for use in this program. These include the "Quality of Life" Scale (QL Scale), the "Symptoms Checklist," and the "Daily Wellness" Check (DW Check). Choose the one (or two or three) that best fits your personal style. Copies of these self-assessment formats are presented here for your initial experimentation. An additional copy of each is found in Appendix E. You may photocopy the format(s) you select to use on a weekly basis and complete the forms as you begin each of the subsequent chapters.

The QL Scale requires 5 minutes to complete. It needs to be completed weekly. The QL Scale includes 17 questions. The questions address two important themes in developing a high quality of life: Emotional Experience and Behavioral Action. As you progress through the exercises in this book, you will see changes in both of these areas. In the area of Emotional Experience, you will become more aware and more accepting. Your feelings may intensify temporarily and then decrease in intensity. Overtime, your ability to tolerate difficult feelings will improve.

Behavioral Action involves two areas. The first concerns your frequency of "Using Coping Strategies" suggested in this book. Your ratings in these areas will increase as you read about the strategies and implement suggested exercises. The second section in the Behavioral Action area involves "Living Your Values" in seven key areas of daily living. We feel more genuine and contented when we "live our values" on a day-to-day basis. The QL Scale asks you to rate the extent to which your behavior reflects your values in each of the key areas. Your scores in the "Behavioral Action" area will increase as you work through this book and your day-to-day behavior aligns more closely with your values.

Try completing the QL Scale now. Use the past week as your reference. Another copy is presented in Appendix E. You may make additional photocopies as needed to evaluate your progress.

The "Symptoms Checklist" offers a second approach to assessment. This method is useful when you are experiencing significant problems with depression. Depression is a somewhat

Quality of Life Scale

Emotional Experience

1. Are you experiencing any of the following feelings on a *daily* basis?

   ☐ Sadness   ☐ Anger   ☐ Fear

2. How intense is your experience of the feelings you checked above? Use this rating scale:

1	2	3	4	5	6	7	8	9	10

   Not Intense   *Very Intense*

3. How willing are you to have the feelings you are having? Use this rating scale:

1	2	3	4	5	6	7	8	9	10

   I cannot tolerate this   *I accept this feeling*
   feeling   *completely*

Behavioral Action

Using Coping Strategies

During the past week, how often have you used the following coping skills? Use this rating scale:

   0 = Not at all   1 = Once   2 = Several times   3 = Almost daily   4 = Daily

1. ___   Participating in pleasurable activities
1. ___   Participating in activities that boost your confidence
1. ___   Simply being aware of an uncomfortable thought, feeling, or emotion without struggling with it
1. ___   Participating in activities that help you relax
1. ___   Using problem-solving techniques for problems you're having in life such as problems with your job or relationships
1. ___   Noticing negative thoughts and replacing them with more realistic thoughts
1. ___   Participating in creative activities

Living Your Values

Please record a number beside each activity to indicate how much you "lived your values" in that area during the past week. Use this rating scale:

1	2	3	4	5	6	7	8	9	10

   Did Not Live What I   *Lived According to My*
   Value   *Values*

1. ___   Enjoying Things Alone   5. ___   Sensual Experience
1. ___   Accomplishing Things Alone   1. ___   Fun with Others
1. ___   Talking with Others   1. ___   Images of a Better Future
1. ___   Contentment with Work

common response to difficult problems of living. Strategies in this book will help you lessen symptoms of depression. Take a moment to complete the checklist now. Use the *past two weeks* as a reference for your answers. You may make additional photocopies for coming weeks from the copy in Appendix E.

If 5 or more of the symptoms on this checklist have been problematic for you more days than not during the past two weeks, you may want to use this method of self-assessment along with the QL Scale. Additionally, you may want to explore use of antidepressant medications in conjunction with this book. Appendix B includes a brief summary of information that may be useful if you are considering medications. Appendix C presents a form for you to complete and take to an appointment with your physician or nurse if you are interested in medications. Appendix D suggests several strategies for using antidepressant medications successfully. If you do start antidepressant therapy, the Symptoms Checklist will help you monitor your response to antidepressant treatment as well as behavioral treatment.

Symptoms Checklist

Please put a check mark by any of the following that have been a problem for you more days than not during the past two weeks.

1. ☐ Anger or Irritability – often during the day
1. ☐ Sadness – often during the day
1. ☐ Sleep Problems: ☐ too much; ☐ slow to go to sleep; ☐ waking in middle of night; ☐ early morning waking
1. ☐ Interest Problems – a lack of interest in others and in activities I usually enjoy
1. ☐ Guilt, self critical thoughts, feeling inadequate or worthless
1. ☐ Energy Problems – tired most of the time
1. ☐ Concentration Problems
1. ☐ Appetite Change: ☐ significantly greater; ☐ significantly less; ☐ weight loss; ☐ weight gain
1. ☐ Psychomotor Problems: ☐ feeling very "slowed down" or ☐ very "speeded up"
1. ☐ More Aches and Pains
1. ☐ Suicidal thoughts

The "Daily Wellness" Check (DW Check) is a third approach to self-assessment. While this approach requires your daily attention, you can complete it quickly and without using any forms. The DW Check may be recorded in a small pocket notebook or a personal calendar. In this approach, you simply record the date and a rating to represent your quality of life. Use a scale of 1 to 10. A rating of 1 means that you "did not live life well." A rating of 10 means that you "lived life well."

You may also want to write down any *positive* thoughts that come to mind at the time when you review your day. You may notice that you have many "ups and downs" during the day. That is normal. Make your daily rating an "average" for the overall day. After you make your rating, record positive thoughts or coping strategies associated with the better moments of your life that day. Look at the example of the Daily Wellness Check.

Daily Wellness Check
Date   **February 4th**
Rate your quality of life today. Record positive thoughts or coping strategies associated with the better moments of your life today.   1   2   3   4   5   6   7   (8)   9   10   *Did not live life well*   *Lived life well*
Thoughts or Activities Related to Rating
1. I had a good sleep last night.
2. This morning I thought, "I will get over this."
3. At lunch, I sat in the sunshine and ate peach ice cream—low fat.
4. I called an old friend after work.

Use the format on the next page to try rating your day as it has been up to this moment. What key thoughts or activities led to your rating for today? You can purchase a small pocket notebook to use for recording your daily wellness information. You may carry it with you throughout the day or simply keep it on a table near your bed. Alternatively, you may want to record daily wellness information in your personal calendar, if you keep one.

You may choose to complete any one or a combination of these three methods of assessment. **If you are very busy and want to complete only one, choose the "Daily Wellness Check."** This approach helps you maintain a daily focus on your life, requires little time, and provides valuable information to guide your behavioral health planning efforts.

Strategies: Generating Hope and Making a Behavioral Health Plan

Two strategies are important this week. The first strategy concerns your sense of optimism. The second strategy involves a method for planning and engaging in behaviors to create more experiences of wellness in your daily life. According to Dr. Aaron Beck (1979), a lack of positive motivation is usually accompanied by a strong desire to avoid constructive activity. Unfortunately, depression and dissatisfaction with life often steer one away from the very activities that would help the most. We may see ourselves as unable to actually perform the activity or we may predict that engaging in the activity would not really be helpful. Hopefulness is a good predictor of action and action is a good predictor of mood change. This chapter helps you address both "hope" and "action" in your life

In 1931, Dr. Alfred Adler said, "Meanings are not determined by situations, but we determine ourselves by the meanings we give to situations (p. 14)." Finding hope for a better future requires you to reconsider the meaning you are giving to current circumstances that trouble you. When you see misfortune as determining your future, your plans for the future may be much more limited than need be. Adversity may provide opportunities to learn new and creative ways of living. Finding "hope" for a better future empowers you to make effective "Behavioral Health Plans." Hope fuels energy to assess, plan, and behave in *new* ways.

Daily Wellness Check		
Date		

Rate your quality of life for today. Record positive thoughts or coping strategies associated with the better moments of your life today.

```
1    2    3    4    5    6    7    8    9    10
```
Did not live life well   *Lived life well*

Thoughts or Activities Related to Rating

1.

2.

3.

4.

Your explanation of your difficulties may enhance or erode your optimism. For example, Marilyn was dissatisfied with her marriage. She saw herself as weak and disgusting for not changing her marriage or leaving her husband. She felt humiliated. She tried to hide from her self-critical interpretation. She did not allow herself to think through her choices. She also tried to hide from others, including a few friends who, incidentally, might have supported her in changing her difficult situation. Dr. Albert Bandura (1977) suggests that there is a reciprocal-interaction between thoughts and behavior. If Marilyn revises her explanation, she may feel more hopeful. For example, she might decide that she is fatigued from the long-term problems in her marriage. Alternatively, she might view herself as simply lacking the skills for getting "unstuck." These alternative views are actually more supported by scientific studies of human behavior. Furthermore, they may have a positive influence on Marilyn's behavior. Endorsement of these revised explanations may encourage her to engage in restorative activities and in a thoughtful re-evaluation of her communication, problem-solving and planning skills.

Making strategic changes in your daily routine usually improves your outlook. It is a mistake to wait until you "*feel*" like doing things that would be good for you. If you succeed in changing your behavior, new thoughts and feelings will follow. **Inspiration comes from doing.**

No one intentionally creates a lousy life. Most of us are attempting to live good lives. Stress overload and use of ineffective strategies block our efforts to live well. If you are blaming or criticizing yourself, stop. With a self-respectful explanation of your present circumstance and a little hope, you will make a plan today to improve your quality of life. Believe in yourself.

Dr. Peter Lewinsohn (1986) suggests specific steps to take to make effective behavioral changes. These steps include assessing problems and planning new life goals. Effective planning requires you to set specific goals and work toward them one small step at a time. Rewarding yourself for your efforts is also important to successful change. Behavioral change is hard work and worthy of positive self-acknowledgment. Finally, close evaluation of the results of having implemented behavioral plans paves the way for on-going constructive action.

Behavioral health planning requires you to be specific, imaginative, observant, and thoughtful. In some cases, behavioral health planning also requires you to ask for feedback from people that you trust. *The more specific the behavioral plans, the easier they are to follow.* For example, a plan to "feel better" or "exercise more" is vague. The starting point is unclear. There is no observable behavior. There is no stated involvement with others. A plan to "walk to the park and back this evening after dinner" is specific. There is a time and place and a behavior that can be *watched*.

At times, your imagination may help you plan creatively. A powerful plan may emerge from a daydream of doing something "different" in your life. Being observant of your thoughts and images during a period of directed fantasy is important. When you are attentive, you may notice "clues" that help you plan more satisfying experiences. Thoughtfulness in planning helps you interrupt your habitual responses to obstacles. There is little value in simply repeating patterns that have not worked for you in the past. Talking your plans over with a trusted friend may also help you turn up new ideas.

Effectiveness: Hoping and Planning

Researchers have found that stress has a less negative impact on people who use active coping strategies (Burns & Nolen-Hoeksema, 1991). Active participation in skill exercises or "homework" is pivotal to success in behavioral change programs. Lazarus (1979) reports that a plan to improve quality of life needs to address numerous areas of one's life. He emphasizes the importance of using several approaches simultaneously to obtain the best results. For example, behavioral plans that address relaxation skills along with interpersonal skills may give a person a stronger opportunity for long-term improvement in quality of life.

I suggest a strategy for self-management called the "Behavioral Health Plan." This method was evaluated in a research study. Over 90% of the people who followed the seven steps in making a "Behavioral Health Plan" went on to implement part or all of the plan. In the next section, I provide information about each of these important steps. In all subsequent chapters, I ask you to use these seven steps to create new plans for your life. Good planning is the key to good follow-through. Remember, your Behavioral Health Plan does not have to result in your "feeling better." For now, limit your focus to forming and implementing the plan. Good plans may take days or even weeks to yield a positive impact on your quality of life.

Generating hope for your future and persistently applying the seven steps of effective behavioral health planning are critical building blocks for living life well. Research findings suggest that people who learn to develop behavioral health plans, review problem-solving skills, and learn to work with their minds and bodies are rewarded with a higher quality of life within one month of concerted effort. Believe in this program, and commit to it.

Goal Setting

Use the questions in the Goal Setting box to assess your present skills. Mark an "x" on top of the number that represents your goal in each area. Circle the number that represents your present skill level in each area. Set a goal to increase your ratings in each area by one (or more) point(s) during the next week. Your Behavioral Health Plan will help structure your initial efforts to apply these strategies. With practice, your skills will improve.

Skill Work

1. Generating Hope

Sit in a quiet place for a few minutes and consider how you choose to explain your current problems. Do you blame yourself? Remember, you are more *like* everybody else in the world than different. You want a high quality of life. All of us do. You are well-intentioned and worthy of self-respect.

Goal Setting

Stimulating Hope

Rate your *sense of hopefulness* at this moment on this scale.

1   2   3   4   5   6   7   8   9   10
Very Little Hope   *Very Hopeful*

Making Behavioral Health Plans

Rate your *confidence* in your ability to make a behavioral health plan that you can implement on this scale.

1   2   3   4   5   6   7   8   9   10
Very Little Confidence   *Very Confidence*

Decide upon an explanation for your current difficulties that reflects a sense of respect for who you are. You may be stressed or overwhelmed or perhaps you simply do not have the skills you need to overcome challenging circumstances. Overhaul your interpretation so that it reflects your worthiness. Write down your revised explanation here.

Revised Explanation

---

2. **Making a Behavioral Health Plan**

Change is the rule in life. We cannot keep things the same (and we often do not *want* to keep things the same). You can make *intentional* changes by making a "Behavioral Health Plan." There are seven steps involved in making a "Behavioral Health Plan." After reading about these steps, use the form on page 22 to apply the steps to your life.

Step One: Select A Focus.

Choose an area of life that you want to address. Choose an area that you believe you can *change easily* and with some improvement to your mood. Choose 1 of the following 7 areas of life as a focus for your plan.

☐   A) Enjoying Things Alone   ☐   E) Sensual Experience
☐   B) Accomplishing Things Alone   ☐   F) Fun with Others
☐   C) Talking with Others   ☐   G) Images of a Better Future
☐   D) Contentment with Work

A) **"Enjoying Things Alone"** refers to activities you do alone that you usually enjoy or new activities that you predict you will enjoy *alone*. For example, Ann used to enjoy going to movies on Fridays with her adult daughter. On occasion, she went to movies without her daughter because she really enjoyed going to the theater. When her daughter moved to another town, Ann stopped going to the movies. Upon reflection, Ann might predict that going to the movies alone on Friday nights would provide her with an experience of "enjoying a life activity alone."

B) **"Accomplishing Things Alone"** refers to two classes of activities: activities you dislike (e.g., cleaning sinks, weeding the garden, or paying bills) and activities that require skill and effort. In the first category, the pleasure of accomplishment comes from completing the undesirable activity. Of course, you can only enjoy a sense of accomplishment *if you acknowledge yourself* for completing the unattractive task.

In the second category, your sense of achievement derives from the process of developing a skill or talent. Examples of accomplishment activities associated with achievement or mastery include athletic, musical, and other artistic activities. Many of our activities provide us with feelings of accomplishment *and* enjoyment. For example, gardening involves weeding an overgrown bed *and* picking a bouquet of flowers. However, experiences of either pleasure *or* accomplishment tend to dominate many life activities.

C) **"Talking with Others"** refers to activities involving direct interpersonal interaction. We are interdependent and have a basic need to communicate effectively with those around us. The nature of our interactions with others may be warm and pleasant, humorous, informational, or conflicted. You are likely to see your values reflected in "talking with others" when you see yourself as genuine, expressive, and effective.

D) **"Contentment with Work"** refers to your connection to work activities and your co-workers. You may spend almost half of your waking hours in your work environment. Skillfulness in managing work stress and in achieving a sense of your value as a worker is important to your sense of well-being.

E) **"Sensual Experience"** refers to your awareness and sensitivity to sensory input. This includes being able to fully "smell" a loaf of fresh-baked bread, "feel" the rise of your chest and abdomen when you inhale, or have goose bumps when listening to one of your favorite pieces of music. Our sensory experience is potentially very powerful, and most of us derive a great deal of satisfaction from selected sensory experiences.

F) **"Fun with Others"** is similar to "Enjoying Things Alone" except that these activities need to involve one or more others. The "other" can be a human being or another animal, such as a pet dog, cat or bird. We are born into a group and live our lives in groups. We value our connections with others, as our very survival depends on them. Research shows that being with others provides a powerful boost to our moods.

G) **"Images of a Better Future"** simply means having thoughts and images about you and your life in the future that are pleasant and rewarding. This type of thinking supplies you with the motivation you need to solve problems and pursue personal goals. Ultimately, most of us value realism and optimism. We need to believe that we can create a better future for ourselves and our loved ones.

Step Two: Imagine.

Imagine yourself doing something that represents your values in one of the seven areas of life. For example, you may value "self-care." If you choose "Contentment with Work" for your Behavioral Health Plan, you may imagine buying a bottle of hand lotion for your desk at work. If you chose "Fun with Others" as your target, you might imagine yourself calling a friend to plan an outing to a baseball game, a restaurant, or a museum. Engaging in this plan reflects a value of sharing enjoyable experiences with others. If you value planning ahead, you may focus on "Images of a Better Future." Consistent with this target and value, you might plan a specific time to think through your lifestyle and make a list of activities you want to incorporate into a better style of living.

Step Three: Plan the Specifics.

Plan a specific time and place to engage in a specific activity that represents "living your values more" in the area of life you decide to address. Vague plans are easy to forget. You need to choose a *distinct* activity and a time to do it, e.g. going bowling on Saturday evening, calling your sister tonight, writing a memo this morning, etc. Choose the day and time of day when you plan to engage in a specific activity. When that time comes, *do it*. Be prepared to implement the plan, even if you are tired or not in the mood, etc. Often, you are more likely to complete the plan if you *mark it on your calendar*, as you would a doctor's appointment.

Step Four: Do It and Observe.

Engage in the planned activity and watch what happens – inside you (*your thoughts, feelings and behaviors*) and outside of you (*what others say or do*). Think of yourself as a scientist and observe carefully. Your observations will help you accurately evaluate results. Be prepared to see results you do not expect. Be open.

Step Five: Reflect.

Think about your findings or results. Ponder your results immediately and again after several hours or days have passed. This is an important aspect of living life well. Too much of the time, we are rushing. Take time to reflect and evaluate your outcomes. For example, a woman made a plan to ask her husband to care for their children for a half hour while she went for a walk. When she asked, her husband agreed *and* showed some irritation with the request. She noted his crankiness and thought of it briefly during the walk. She considered returning home after two blocks. Then, she intentionally shifted her focus to gardens and houses she saw. She noted the colors and texture of plants. She breathed deeply and hummed one of her favorite tunes. When she returned from the walk, she felt refreshed. She felt grateful for the time alone, and she thanked her husband. He seemed relaxed at that point. Later in the evening, he told her that he was glad that she went for her walk. In reflecting on the implementation of her plan, she realized the importance of *watching her responses* during the plan. This step of "watching" helped her continue with the plan rather than turning back early. "Watching" also helped her realize that her husband's displeasure with the request was temporary.

Step Six: Discuss.

Talk with others about your results and draw conclusions. The woman in the example above talked with a friend about her Behavioral Health Plan and concluded that she would continue with her requests for her husband to watch the children while she went for a walk in the evening. Further, she concluded that she did not need to concern herself with her husband's testiness, as it appeared to be short-lived and not representative of his desire to support her.

Step Seven: Plan Further.

Make another Behavior Health Plan. This is a very important step. In order to live life well, you do need to continue to plan and to change when plans do not work well.

Use the "Making a Behavioral Health Plan Exercise" format to develop your initial plan. Review the example as well.

Making a Behavioral Health Plan: An Exercise	
Steps	**Plan**
1. Choose an area of life that you want to address.	
2. Imagine yourself doing something that represents your values in that area of life.	
3. Plan a specific time and place to engage in specific activity.	
4. Engage in the planned activity and watch what happens inside and outside of you.	
5. Think about your findings or results.	
6. Talk with others about your results and draw conclusions.	
7. Make another behavioral health plan.	

Example: Hoping and Planning

James was a high school teacher and a father of three. He experienced several life changes in a two-year period that had a negative impact on his sense of well-being. His wife returned to full time work several months after his best friend moved forty miles away. He had a change in his teaching schedule, which required him to work more hours. Finally, he suffered a knee injury that interfered with his usual daily jog of 2 or 3 miles. James felt discouraged and cranky. He was sleeping poorly and overeating at times. He watched television more than he wanted, but needed "an escape."

James selected "Enjoying Things Alone" as the area of life to target in his plan. In that he valued good health, he imagined engaging in a physical activity that he enjoyed and that would promote good physical and mental health. James decided to try swimming. As you can see in the skill work example, James developed a specific plan to go to his community pool and pick up a schedule on Monday and to swim one day after work during the week. As indicated on the skill worksheet, James felt apprehensive when he arrived at the pool, but relaxed after his swim. Because he was observant of what happened "outside" as well as "inside" when he engaged in the planned activity, he noticed that his wife greeted him with more affection than usual after his swim. James concluded that swimming was within his physical capabilities and had a positive impact on his mood. He discussed his health plan with his physician and decided to swim three times each week for the next month.

Making a Behavioral Health Plan: An Example	
Steps	**Plan**
1. Choose an area of life that you want to address.	Enjoying Things Alone.
2. Imagine yourself doing something that represents your values in that area of life.	Swimming.
3. Plan a specific time and place to engage in specific activity.	Go to the Community pool on Monday after work and pick up a schedule; plan one time to swim after work during the next week.
4. During and after the experiment, watch what happens inside and outside of you.	Inside: Felt worried about my appearance at the pool. Very little pain in knee during the swim. Felt relaxed and "at peace" after swimming. Outside: Wife gave me a kiss when I came home after swimming.
5. Think about your findings or results.	I am physically capable of swimming and it improves my mood.
6. Talk with others about your results and draw conclusions.	Talked with my primary care physician at a check-up on my knee. Physician was supportive of my continuing to swim.
7. Make another behavioral health plan.	Swim three times per week for the next month.

Behavioral Health Plan: Hoping and Planning

Use the Behavioral Health Plan form at the end of this chapter to summarize the details of your first plan. The Behavioral Health Plan has two sections. The first asks you to revise your interpretation of a current problem so that you feel more hopeful. The second section helps you summarize the details of your first behavioral change plan. Complete these two sections now.

Reinforce your efforts by rewarding yourself. Changing your behavior is hard work. Plan a small reward for yourself–buying or picking a fresh flower for your dining table, watching a football game on Monday night, scheduling a mini-massage. Record your planned reward on the planning format.

Your commitment to the plan is essential. If you cannot commit 100% to your plan, revise it now so that it merits more of your confidence. When you have more confidence in your plan, you will be able to muster commitment. For example, Elizabeth originally planned to go to bed and read a magazine at 10:00 PM. When she assessed her commitment level, she realized that she would struggle with skipping certain late evening tasks such as tidying her kitchen and making school lunches for her children. She revised her plan to start reading in bed at 10:30 and felt more confident and committed.

If you do not implement your Behavioral Health Plan as written during the next week, make note of what part or parts of the plan *you did* implement and what interfered with the plan's full implementation. Working with a friend, therapist, nurse, or physician may help you be more successful. I encourage you to enlist the support of another person before moving to Chapter 2.

References

Adler, A. (Ed.). (1931). *What life should mean to you*. New York: Capricorn, 1958.

Bandura, A. *Social learning theory*. Englewood Cliffs, N.J.: Prentice Hall, 1977.

Beck, A. T., Rush, A. J., Shaw, B. F., & Emery, G. (1979). *Cognitive Therapy of Depression*. New York, NY: The Guilford Press.

Burns, D.D., & Nolen-Hoeksema, S. (1991). Coping styles, homework compliance, and the effectiveness of cognitive-behavioral therapy. *Journal of Consulting and Clinical Psychology, 59*(2), 305-311.

Katon, W., Robinson, P., Von Korff, M., Lin, E., Bush, T., Ludman, E., Simon, G., & Walker, E. (1996). A multifaceted intervention to improve treatment of depression in primary care. *Archives of General Psychiatry, 53*(10), 924-932.

Lazarus, A. (1990). The multimodal approach to the treatment of minor depression. *American Journal of Psychotherapy, XIV* (1), 50-57.

Lewinsohn, P. M., Ricardo, F. M., Youngren, M. A., & Zeiss, A. M. (1986). *Control your depression*. New York: Prentice Hall Press.

Robinson, P. (1995). New territory for the behavior therapist . . . hello, depressed patients in primary care. *The Behavior Therapist*, September.

Robinson, P., Bush, T., Von Korff, M., Katon, W., Lin, W., Simon, G. E., & Walker, E. (1995). Primary care physician use of cognitive behavioral techniques with depressed patients. *Journal of Family Practice, 40*(4), 352-357.

Robinson, P., Katon, W., Von Korff, M., Bush, T., Ludman, E., Simon, G., Lin, E., & Walker, E. (1996). Use of coping strategies by depressed primary care patients: Results of a randomized controlled trial. Submitted for publication.

Behavioral Health Plan
Building Hope And Planning To Improve Life

How do you explain your present difficulties?

Does this explanation assume that you are a creative person worthy of respect from yourself and others?   ☐ Yes   ☐ No

If needed, revise your explanation so it reflects the assumption that you are a person worthy of respect.

Does your revised explanation have a positive impact on your hopefulness?   ☐ Yes ☐ No

The area of life I will target in my plan this week is:

☐ Enjoying Things Alone   ☐ Sensual Experience

☐ Accomplishing Things Alone   ☐ Fun with Others

☐ Talking with Others   ☐ Images of a Better Future

☐ Contentment with Work

I plan to:

I will do this when:

I will do this where:

I will do this with whom:

Who will support my plan?

As a reward for following my Behavioral Health Plan, I will:

Am I 100% committed to this Plan?   ☐ Yes   ☐ No

Chapter 2

Building Acceptance And Making Value-Based Choices

Weekly Review

Last week, you revised your explanation of your present difficulties. You tried to make your explanation consistent with the assumption that you are a good person who is capable of living life creatively and intelligently. Did a shift in your interpretation have a positive impact on your mood? Do you feel more confident in yourself and/or more positive about other people in your life? Rate your sense of hopefulness and your self-confidence in making behavioral health plans at the present moment.

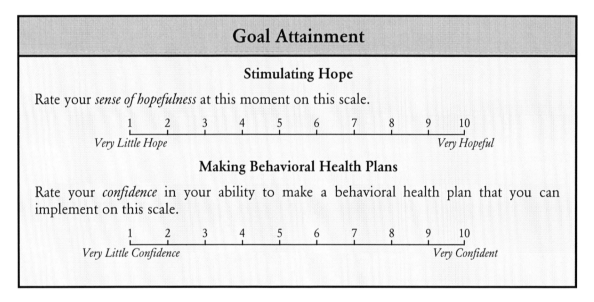

Compare your present Goal Attainment ratings with your Goal Setting ratings in Chapter 1. Is your hopefulness rating higher? Are there any specific activities or thoughts that tend to enhance your sense of optimism? What are they?

Did your confidence in your ability to make and implement a behavioral health plan improve? Did the plan have a positive impact on your sense of wellness? What obstacles did you encounter? If you had difficulties in formulating *or* implementing your plan, you may want to review Chapter 1 now.

Behavioral health planning involves numerous skills. It is a basic strategy in creating a lifestyle that reflects your values. Formulating effective behavioral change plans requires skill and practice. At present, measure your success by the extent to which you *followed the steps* suggested in Chapter 1. If your plans do not have a positive impact on your mood soon, you may want to involve a health care professional in your behavioral change program. If you are already working with a health care professional, discuss your results with them.

Self-Assessment

Complete the method(s) of self-assessment that you choose to use in tracking your progress. You may photocopy the assessment form(s) most useful to you from Appendix E. **If you are using the Quality of Life Scale** (QL Scale), do your present ratings differ from your last ratings? If so, examine the differences. Of particular interest, did your Behavioral Health Plan have an impact on your ability to express your values in the area of life targeted by the plan? Often, a Behavioral Health Plan will boost expression of values in several life areas, as there is a spill-over effect. For example, Lisa planned to go to dinner with a group of friends in an effort to improve expression of her value of socializing with others. She targeted the area of having "Fun with Others." Her ratings improved slightly in "Fun with Others" *and* "Accomplishment Alone." Lisa drove alone to an unknown area of the city in order to meet her friends. This was somewhat difficult for her, and she remembered to acknowledge herself for pushing through this potential obstacle to her plan.

What did you notice inside and outside of yourself while you implemented your plan? Did you notice uncomfortable sensations? Tension? Sadness? Self-critical thoughts? Self-doubting thoughts? Fearful images? On the inside, Lisa noticed thoughts of becoming lost, being late, and being inadequate. She noticed images of being laughed at by her friends, and sensations of increased shoulder and neck tension, sweating, and pressure on her throat and chest. On the outside, she noticed that she arrived safely and was greeted warmly by her friends. As she relaxed, she conversed easily with several people and actually enjoyed her dinner. Finally, Lisa evaluated her results. She evaluated her plan and decided to plan *more* social outings. She planned to have coffee with a co-worker three days after the dinner outing. Additionally, she called her sister in another state for a long phone visit.

If you are using the Symptoms Checklist, compare your present responses with your original responses. Are there changes? Where are your improvements? Both behavioral strategies and medications may help lessen symptoms of depression. Persevere and change will come.

If you are using the Daily Wellness Check, what were your highest and lowest daily ratings during the past week? How did these two days differ? What key thoughts or activities are associated with your days when you "live well?" Do you see any themes or behavioral patterns emerging? For example, Ed noticed a tendency to engage in a lot of self-evaluative thought when he arrived at work in the morning. On better days, he tended to acknowledge himself as a creative and persistent worker in the mornings and to complete a small difficult task prior to his morning break. Take a moment to reflect and write down a few examples of thoughts and activities in your life that are associated with higher quality experiences in your day-to-day life.

Discoveries from Daily Wellness Checks During the Past Week
1.
2.
3.
4.

Strategies: Building Acceptance and Making Value-Based Choices

Psychological acceptance is a coping strategy that enables you to embrace, rather than struggle with, obstacles to living life well. When you can embrace rather than resist obstacles, you can change your behavior. Everyone faces obstacles to living in accordance with important values. For instance, we all have unwanted thoughts and feelings. Your personal history determines the specific personal barriers you encounter in living according to your intentions. To a great extent, we cannot control whether we have "issues," "weak spots" or "skeletons in the closet." What we can control is the decision to move ahead in life. This requires that we acknowledge our weaknesses.

Psychological acceptance empowers you to engage in committed action. It is the active process of embracing obstacles and accepting them as "challenges." It enables you to make value-based choices in life. Value-based choices are decisions that reflect what you believe to be truly important in life. Psychological acceptance is a foundation stone for all of the strategies presented in this book.

I will give you a concrete example of psychological acceptance in action. I am looking for the scissors, and I shut my finger in a drawer. My young child is watching me look for the scissors because we plan to wrap a present together. My finger is throbbing and turning purple. I can respond in a number of ways. I could swear at the drawer. Alternatively, I could sit on the floor, hold my painful finger, and take slow, deep breaths. The appeal of swearing at the drawer is that it gives me a chance to "right the wrong." Unfortunately, this option would lead me personally into another value conflict. I value solving problems without profanity and I want to demonstrate this belief to my child who is watching me closely. If I go with my urge to swear, I feel guilty. The guilt feels really rotten, so I could look for a way to move away psychologically from this discomfort. Since my child is still standing there, I could blame her. I could suggest that she probably neglected to put the scissors away. Further, I could tell her that she should not be talking to me when I am looking for the scissors. I could top it off by announcing, "I do not even want to wrap the present anymore." This spiral escalates easily and may be appropriately called the "struggle spin out." The alternative of being fully present with the initial pain of an injured finger is difficult because it requires an action that differs from our usual patterns. Most of us are accustomed to taking action toward or away from someone or something when we are hurting physically or psychologically.

Psychological acceptance involves taking action *toward the self*. It requires active acceptance of personal experience. When we embrace our experience, we are able to make qualitatively different decisions about our behavior. In returning to the above example, my behavioral choice after accepting my pain might simply be to get ice for my finger and rest a while.

Many problems of living may be addressed by using psychological acceptance methods. In 1994, Steven Hayes explained how psychological acceptance strategies can promote a general sense of wellness. He suggested five common targets for on-going practice of psychological acceptance and committed behavioral actions. These obstacles will seem familiar to you, as all are basic to the human predicament.

1. **Non-acceptance of self.** All of us have anxieties and fears. We question our worth, our adequacy, our ability to be loved. We may spend years trying to control uncomfortable thoughts and feelings about our "self." Numerous people turn to alcohol or other drugs to escape painful, negative thoughts of self. The dilemma is this: Negative thoughts about yourself are painful *and* you cannot get rid of negative thoughts about yourself.

    Behavioral change methods may help you temporarily *lessen* distressing thoughts about yourself. However, they cannot help you *eliminate* negative thoughts about yourself on a long-term basis. Behavioral change methods enable you to suppress self-critical thoughts about yourself, and, *suppression is a short-term solution.* Suppressed thoughts often return "energized" in the *very near future.*

    Positive and negative thoughts and images of the self are a part of human experience. They require exploration. If you take the time to examine painfully negative thoughts about yourself, you become more familiar with them. You can even learn to have a "friendly" response to recurring negative thoughts. You can learn to say, "Hi, there. I know you, my self-doubting thoughts." Unconditional self-acceptance is the ground work for solid emotional and behavioral health (Ellis, 1990). Self-respect grows from acceptance of your own unique, personal thoughts, images, sensations, and feelings–both negative and positive.

Self-respect cannot be earned by good deeds *or* from positive evaluations of others. *Only you* can give yourself self-respect. Given the on-going nature of negative thoughts about self, you need to give yourself the gift of self-respect *again and again* in life. You started giving yourself self-respect last week when you formulated an explanation of your current difficulties that assumed your inherent worth *and* your potential expertise on living life well. Having negative and critical self-statements does not contradict your gift of self-respect when you respond to your negative self-statements for what they are–*just thoughts, not truths.*

Negative self-statements are thoughts from your past triggered by your present difficult experiences. The negative self-statements often have no real application to the present challenges you are facing. Furthermore, energy you spend struggling with these negative thoughts is energy you do not have for solving *current* problems of living. Negative self-statements are free to come and go when you respond to them with openness rather than struggle. When you can accept painfully critical thoughts about yourself, you are in the position to choose your actions. Your choice evolves from *what you value and what needs to be done* in your life at the present moment.

For example, Mary's father died when she was young. Her mother struggled with accepting this loss. She was critical of Mary when she grieved for her father. As an adult, Mary experienced considerable stress in response to any type of loss. She tended to feel vulnerable and depressed. She habitually withdrew from her friends when she was confronted with even minor losses. Mary found the idea of psychological acceptance intriguing. When she began to practice acceptance exercises, she noticed a flood of self-disparaging thoughts when she felt lonely or sad. Overtime, she learned to experience her self-critical thoughts and her sad feelings gracefully. In the more gentle context of psychological acceptance, these thoughts were less provocative. Mary was more able to pursue use of behavioral change plans based on her values and identity as an adult. She valued friendship and open expression of feelings. Therefore, she began to express her sense of loss in response to specific situations to one of her close friends. The friend responded with interest and support. Mary accepted painful thoughts about herself. She was then empowered to change her behavior and her life moved forward.

2. **Avoidance of Situations.** Often, we avoid situations in an effort to control unwanted thoughts, feelings and sensations. Contact with certain people or places or participation in specific activities may provoke unwanted thoughts, feelings, or sensations. Avoidance strategies can be helpful on a short-term basis. However, avoidance proves disruptive when employed as a basic control strategy. One's life becomes "smaller and smaller" when avoidance becomes a dominant style for controlling unwanted thoughts and feelings.

Most of us have had the experience of engaging in meaningless behavior arising from an effort to avoid unwanted thoughts and feelings. You probably remember the childhood rhyme, "Step on a crack and you break your mother's back." Today, you probably can say, "That's ridiculous." However, can you instruct yourself, "Step on a crack and break your mother's back," and step on one sidewalk crack after another *and* remain open to your psychological experience? Most of us would probably prefer to avoid the cracks or find a distraction rather than experience the increasing tension associated with behaving in a way that "breaks a language rule" implying willful harm to our mother. The extent to which you can step on the cracks and willingly experience your personal responses represents your ability to apply a psychological acceptance strategy and "embrace" this troublesome childhood verse.

Let's take a more challenging example. Tom's father was anxious in social situations and managed his discomfort by avoiding social situations altogether when he could and being quiet when avoidance was not an option. Like most adults, Tom patterned his behavior after his father to some extent. He reasoned, "If I am quiet or stay home, I will not feel anxious." As an adult, he implemented this strategy steadfastly to no avail. He felt anxious when he talked with others, when he was quiet, when he stayed home, and when he went out into the world. Avoiding interaction with others and social gatherings only added to his anxiety as he spent a great deal of time *anticipating* unwanted interactions. Practicing psychological acceptance techniques helped Tom to enter risky social situations where he could experience a range of feelings, including happiness, sadness, anxiety, and well-being. When you enter into previously avoided situations, your actual experience will usually differ from what you expect. Tom found that he enjoyed talking with people who had similar interests. He valued being outdoors. With continued practice of psychological acceptance, he joined a bird-watching club.

Mark is another example of a person attempting to control unwanted feelings though psychological avoidance. Mark was a 38 year old drafter. He could not be around his parents and brothers without consuming alcoholic beverages. He anticipated that he "just could not take the family" without a drink first. When he did expose himself to his family without drinking, he noticed that other family members teased him about abstaining and that he became angry in a conversation with two of his brothers. Also, he noticed that his anger passed without expression and that his tension lessened over time. He actually enjoyed the cranberry juice he drank at the family party and felt good the next morning.

3. **An Impulse to Be "Right."** When was the last time you had the unpleasant experience of trying to persuade someone to change her/his behavior because you knew the "right" way to behave. "Being right" is frequently a theme in work conflicts and in conflicts with intimates as well. In some cases, a person will sacrifice a relationship, or even, his or her life, to "be right."

    Psychological acceptance helps you acknowledge an "I am right and you are wrong" agenda. The act of "embracing" the agenda empowers you to step out of the injunction to be "right." You can evaluate the ultimate importance of a particular issue relative to the potential damage done to the relationship if you pursue being "right." You can choose between implementing the "be right" agenda at the level of behavior *or* simply "noticing" the psychological presence of the "be right" agenda *and behaving according to your values*. Often, a particular issue is not as important as the continuation of a respectful relationship on a longer-term basis.

    For example, Kirk had a conflict with his new supervisor regarding his service to a long-standing account. The supervisor was new and lacked the experience that Kirk had in working with these particular customers. While Kirk wanted to "be right," he valued the development of a good relationship with his new supervisor more than "winning" on this issue. Kirk used psychological acceptance to *make room* for his personal, private experience of angry thoughts and feelings. His anger passed without contaminating the new working relationship and, over time, the supervisor gave more credence to Kirk's opinions.

4. **Wanting a "Recipe" for Living.** Recipes work well in the kitchen and less well elsewhere. Mastery of many life activities comes only through a series of trials *and errors*. Many parents probably want to write down the rules of love for their teenagers. Wise is the parent who gives up early on the rule approach and simply encourages teenage children to "*Let your experience be your teacher.*" In a similar vein, you may have noticed shy children or been one yourself. The timid person may seek "rules" to follow in learning skills such as public speaking. While some verbal instructions and modeling are useful, nothing can measure up to the learning potential inherent in direct experience.

As an adult, you may look for self-help books to give you a "recipe" on how to respond to stressful life transitions. For example, you may long for more instruction on how to behave in a new marriage, when you have a baby or when you care for an aging parent. Guide books may be helpful. However, an over-reliance on rules in solving particular life problems may lead you to be less sensitive to subtle information. When you are exceedingly reliant on rules, you may continue to apply rules even when they work poorly in a specific situation. You may even apply the rules more steadfastly when your experience tells you that the recipe is not solving the current dilemma. When you can accept the failure of "cherished rules," you are more able to detect small, subtle changes in a situation that relate to your behavior efforts. Detection of these effects can lead you to exhibit other *new behaviors* in a currently challenging area of your life. Psychological acceptance can enable you to accept the limits of a "recipe," embrace the moment and trust your direct experience of *what works for you for now in this context*.

When you go by your experience, you can never be wrong. Your experience is always exactly *as it is*. Rules will always be less accurate than your experience. Psychological acceptance helps you perceive a "collection of rules" in your own mind or notice a "recipe request" in someone else's mind, while focusing on your experience and the priceless lessons attending direct experience.

5. **Protesting Fairness.** You probably learned language about "fairness" around the age of four or five. Roughly speaking, "This is not fair" means this is not going the way I want it to go. Resolution of fairness issues is possible through compromise when the events of concern can be influenced or changed. When the event or situation is unchangeable, protesting fairness can get one "stuck" in feeling resentful and sad. We often cling to our anger because we see it as our "right." Unfortunately, time spent in anger, righteousness, or self-pity is time lost to more effective, present-oriented problem-solving strategies. Further, prolonged anger is stressful to the body.

Fairness disputes are common in close relationships. For example, Lynn and Bill were struggling in their marriage of four years. Lynn had always wanted Bill to be more emotionally expressive. She had used different change-oriented techniques to try to improve his disclosure of feelings, etc. Lynn modeled emotional expression, as this came quite easily for her. She hoped that her example and her repeated requests would change Bill. Unfortunately, Bill valued his ability to deal with his emotional experience privately. Lynn's efforts to change him triggered his urge to "dig his heels in" and be even more unflappable. When Lynn used psychological acceptance strategies, she was able to accept her own emotional experience. Lynn came to realize that she felt painfully "*alone and helpless*" when Bill was upset and withdrew from her. Accepting her "aloneness" and "helplessness" allowed her to change her behavior. She had an opportunity to behave according to her values. She did not value "controlling her spouse." She valued taking care of herself and "being open" to her spouse. Lynn decided to reflect these values in her behavior. When Bill withdrew, she started to "check in" with herself. She learned to experience her own angst about this difference between herself and her spouse, and, then, to engage in personally satisfying activities (e.g., listening to music). She remained open to Bill and responded with warmth when he approached her.

Psychological acceptance can assist you in responding to unwanted and unchangeable events such as death of a loved one or loss of physical health due to accidental injury or catastrophic illness. When you accept these types of painful life experiences fully, you are less likely to be "thrown off" your course by similar unfortunate events in the future. Practicing acceptance skills is well worth your time, as life presents us with more and more opportunities to respond to unwanted, unchangeable events and circumstances as we age.

Effectiveness: Psychological Acceptance

Psychological acceptance is an effective approach to coping with unwanted thoughts, feelings, and images. Excessive use of alcohol and other psychoactive drugs, depression and anxiety-related conditions, and certain interpersonal problems (for example, strong dependency) are examples of problems that respond well to acceptance techniques. Kabat-Zinn and his colleagues (1992) reported that participation in a mindfulness meditation class helped participants reduce symptoms of anxiety and panic. Patients with generalized anxiety and panic maintained reductions over time.

Hayes and Strosahl (1996) presented evidence concerning the effectiveness of acceptance strategies with depression. Strategies were particularly helpful concerning experience of distressing suicidal ideation. A researcher in Great Britain, Dr. John Teasdale, also provided information about use of mindfulness training in depression treatment and prevention of future episodes of depression.

Another British researcher found that a combination of acceptance-related strategies (30 minutes of yogic stretching and breathing exercises) had an "invigorating" effect on perceptions of mental and physical energy in a group of adults aged 21 to 76. Additionally, the exercises resulted in more positive mood states (Wood, 1993). Of course, acceptance approaches help you heal from unchangeable events, including psychologically painful experiences in childhood and adulthood and the challenges of normal aging. Older adults who received mindfulness training became healthier and lived longer than older adults not trained in mindfulness (Alexander, et al., 1989).

Psychological acceptance techniques are also associated with improvement in motor skills and ability to cope with illness. In a 1993 study, school children who received 10 days of training in stretching, focusing, and breathing exercises demonstrated performance on a motor task that was superior to children who did not receive training in acceptance strategies (Telles, et al., 1993). Acceptance strategies involving yoga training helped young asthmatics improve significantly in pulmonary function and exercise capacity (Jain, et al., 1991). Further, persons with HIV/AIDS who practiced meditation, which is also a psychological acceptance method, scored higher on measures of mental and physical hardiness than non-meditators (Carson, 1993).

Finally, psychological acceptance is helpful in the difficult process of habit change in general psychotherapy and in therapy for addiction problems. In their book, *Relapse Prevention*, Dr. Allen Marlatt and his colleague, Dr. Gordon, suggested use of metaphors as imagery techniques in coping with urges to relapse or return to use of problematic substances, such as nicotine or alcohol. They draw from a Buddhist scholar, Shunryu Suzuki. Mr. Suzuki offers a metaphor for use in habit change: "To give your sheep or cow a large spacious meadow is the way to control him." People who report eventual, long-term success in giving up smoking or coping with a significant weight problem typically report that their rate of progress was uneven and marked by numerous setbacks (Schachter, 1990). Use of psychological acceptance strategies are highly effective with people who have struggled many years with dependence on alcohol and other psychoactive drugs (Hayes, 1993). Step 11 (or practice of meditation) among participants in the Alcoholics Anonymous Program is significantly correlated with more purpose in life and longer lengths of sobriety (Carrol, 1993). Psychological acceptance strategies have a very wide range of applicability.

Goal Setting

Use the questions in the Goal Setting box to assess your present level of skill in using psychological acceptance skills. Try to increase your ratings in one (or both) of these areas, by one (or more) points during the coming week. Mark you present skill level with a circle around the

---

Goal Setting

I recommend that you set two goals concerning development of psychological acceptance skills.

Focusing Skills

Rate your ability to *focus* on sensations of breathing for 5 minutes at the present moment on this scale.

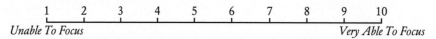

Unable To Focus   Very Able To Focus

Creating the Acceptance Mind State

Rate your confidence in your ability to *create a state of mind* associated with psychological acceptance. Use this scale to rate your ability to "give your mind a large spacious meadow" at the present moment.

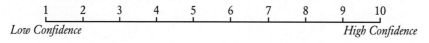

Low Confidence   High Confidence

---

number and your goal with an "x" on the number. After a week of practice you will rate your skills in the Goal Attainment box in Chapter 3. With practice, you can reach your goals.

Skill Work: Identifying, Observing, Accepting

There are five steps in developing basic psychological acceptance skills. This approach to coping may seem awkward to you. It is subtle and requires a great deal of concentration. Use the following steps to cultivate psychological acceptance. Your reward will be *greater consistency* in implementing behavior plans that reflect your values.

Step One: Identify Difficulties.

Identify specific psychological experiences you want to control or avoid. This is a difficult first step. Give it thought and effort. The "Checklist of Intolerable and Restricted Psychological Experiences" on the next page will help you generate an initial list of psychological experiences that make you feel "out of control." *Check items that you consistently find intolerable and actively resist.*

Step Two: Generate Specific Descriptors.

Write out more descriptive information on each item checked above. For example, if you checked "Fear," you might add a description of "feeling sweaty and having my heart pound." For every feeling, thought, image, or event you checked, write out several more descriptive words or phrases on a small piece of paper. You will probably have eight or ten small pieces of paper with experiences you want to avoid. Fold each piece of paper separately and place them in an envelope or bowl.

Step Three: Develop A Method of Self-Observation.

In order to develop more acceptance of difficult psychological phenomena, you need a workable method for *staying aware* and actively maintaining an observing, accepting, attitude. Several sensory approaches are helpful. People differ in sensory preferences, so you will need to

A Checklist of Intolerable and Resisted Psychological Experiences	
Area	**Specific Experience**
1. Feelings	☐ Fear ☐ Anxiety ☐ Panic ☐ Depression ☐ Sadness ☐ Anger ☐ Other:
2. Thoughts	☐ of Aggression ☐ of Self Harm ☐ of Violence ☐ of Death ☐ of Poor Health ☐ of Loss ☐ of Being Rejected ☐ of Being Homeless ☐ of Being Unworthy or Unlovable ☐ of Being Injured or Attacked ☐ of Being Out of Control
3. Images	☐ of Violence ☐ of Helplessness ☐ of Ridicule ☐ Other:

experiment to find a method that works for you. For example, Joanna is a "visual" person and she prefers the support of a visual image in self-observation exercises. Visual methods involve placing the psychological experience you observe onto a visual referent. For example, thoughts, feelings, and images can be allowed to float onto a puff of smoke as they arise in your awareness. Frances, on the other hand, is a more "auditory" person. She prefers verbal instruction to support her self observation. "I have a thought of . . ." or "I have a picture of . . ." are useful verbal or auditory structures for embracing or welcoming psychological phenomena *in the moment.*

Step Four: Use the Breathe–Observe–Stimulate–Embrace (BOSE) Procedure.

The BOSE procedure needs to be carefully followed numerous times during every practice period. This procedure involves the following steps.

Breathe. Take four deep breaths and count as you inhale. With each breath, move further into your "observation" perspective.

Observe. Start the use of your visual or verbal metaphor to structure your focus on psychological phenomena that enter your awareness.

Stimulate. After several minutes of watching, take a piece of paper from your bowl of avoided phenomena. Read the words and continue to hold the paper in your hands.

Embrace. State to yourself, "This thought (feeling, image) is mine. It belongs to me."

Return to the initial BOSE step and proceed through this process again and again during your practice periods. When you "space out," gently bring yourself back to the exercise by recalling the steps involved in the BOSE procedure.

Step Five: Expand Practice to Daily Life.

After a week of daily practice of the BOSE procedure, you may begin to apply psychological acceptance approaches of breathing, using an observational structure (visual or verbal/auditory), and accepting/embracing in daily situations that provoke concerns about control. For example, Rachel began to use the BOSE approach when she felt annoyed by a difficult co-worker. As she became more accepting of her anger (and her "be right" agenda), she became more intentional (and less reactive) in her responses to the on-going problematic relationship. As you approach this step, you may want to make several visual reminders for yourself. You can write out a "cue" on a note card. Additionally, you might plan one or two "BOSE" sessions during your daily routine. In a brief review, you can re-evaluate your psychological experience during the previous 2- to 3-hour period to identify any missed opportunities for applying this subtle yet powerful strategy.

Example: Acceptance and Value-Based Choices

Karen did not accept her husband's consumption of alcohol. Her father had been alcoholic during her childhood and her parents often argued about his drinking. Over the course of the twelve year marriage, her husband drank more and more beer in the evening, and she felt more and more distressed. Karen tried to control her distress by controlling her husband's drinking. She nagged him more and more. Unfortunately, her carping had little impact other than to escalate the marital conflict.

When Karen began to practice psychological acceptance methods, she discovered that she experienced a sense of helplessness and fear when her husband opened a beer. She practiced breathing techniques and worked to accept her frightening thoughts and uncomfortable feelings on a daily basis. At times, she found herself crying during her practice periods. She allowed her tears to come and used the BOSE method to help her accept difficult thoughts and sensations as they arose in her mind and body. Overtime, she was more and more able to tolerate her uncomfortable feelings and associated thoughts of "losing control." Karen began to badger her husband less.

Eventually, Karen made a commitment to respond to her experience of helplessness with behaviors that were more consistent with her desire to live life well. When she noticed fears surfacing in response to her husband's drinking behaviors, she accepted her fear and became more aware of painful thoughts and images from her childhood that she had previously avoided by pestering her husband. After a period of stillness (and BOSE practice), she allowed herself to continue with her usual activities or shift to activities that gave her a sense of calm and pleasure. She set up a comfortable area for knitting in her living room. She went to this special place to experience the fears and memories triggered by her husband's having a beer.

After a month of practice, Karen felt less of a need to stay home in the evening to monitor her husband's drinking and joined a book club, where she made several friends. While her thoughts of being "out of control" did not disappear (where could they go!), *the thoughts controlled her behavior less*. In calm, quiet moments, she began a systematic evaluation of her marriage, which eventually led her to conclude that the marriage was no longer satisfying to her. She asked her husband to re-evaluate his investment in the marriage.

Behavioral Health Plan: Applying Acceptance Strategies

Your Behavioral Health Plan for this week requires you to commit to practice of acceptance strategies. Complete the first section now. The second section involves developing a behavioral change plan. Select one of the seven areas of life. Optimally, you will select an area of life that needs to change in order to better mirror your personal values. This question may help you identify an area of focus: "Which area(s) would need to change in order for you to have a lifestyle that expresses what is most important to you?" Complete the details of a behavioral change plan (i.e., when, where, with whom, and who will support you). If necessary, review Chapter 1 to help you develop a clear and specific plan that merits your confidence and commitment. Also, remember to plan a small reward to encourage you to continue your work in this program. Assess your level of commitment to your plan. If it is not high, change your plan. Make it easier or more specific. The key to effective behavioral change is making realistic plans. Change occurs one small step at a time.

More skillful observation of your mental activities unlocks your potential for making value-based choices. When your behavior is consistent with your values, you experience more well-being in life. Of course, living life well does not mean being free of psychological pain. When we live life well, we have many feelings–some very pleasant and some quite painful.

References

Alexander, C., Langer, E., Newman, R., Chandler, H., & Davies, J. (1989). Transcendental meditation, mindfulness, and longevity: An experimental study with the elderly. *Journal of Personality and Social Psychology, 57,* 950-964.

Carrol, S. (1993). Spirituality and purpose in life in alcoholism recovery. *Journal of Studies on Alcohol, 54*(3), 297-301.

Carson, V. B. (*1993).* Prayer, meditation, exercise, and special diets: Behaviors of the hardy person with HIV/AIDS. *Journal of the Association of Nurses in AIDS Care, 4*(3), 18-28.

Hayes, S. (1994). Content, context, and the types of psychological acceptance. In S. Hayes, N. Jacobson, V. Follette, & M. Dougher (Eds.), *Acceptance and change: Content and context in psychotherapy*, (pp. 13-35). Reno, NV: Context Press.

Hayes, S. (1995). Personal communication.

Hayes, S. C., Strosahl, K. D., & Wilson, K. G. (1999). *Acceptance and commitment therapy: An experiential approach to behavior change.* New York, NY: Guilford Press.

Jain, S. C., Rai, l., Valecha, A., Jha, U.K., Bhatnagar, S. O., & Ram, K. (1991). Effect of yoga training on exercise tolerance in adolescents with childhood asthma. *Journal of Asthma, 28*(6), 437-442.

Kabat-Zinn, J., Massion, A. O., Kristeller, J., Peterson, L. G., Fletcher, K. E., Pbert, L., Lenderking, W. R., & Santorelli, S. F. (1992). Effectiveness of a meditation-based stress reduction program in the treatment of anxiety disorders. *American Journal of Psychiatry, 149*(7), 936-943.

Marlatt, G. A., & Gordon, J. R. (1985). *Relapse prevention: Maintenance strategies in the treatment of addictive behaviors.* New York, NY: Guilford Press.

Schachter, S. (1990). Debunking myths about self-quitting: Evidence from 10 prospective studies of persons who attempt to quit smoking by themselves: Reply. *American Psychologist, 45,* 1389-1390.

Suziki, S. (1970). *Zen mind, beginner's mind.* New York: Weatherhill.

Teasdale, J. D., Segal, Z., & Williams, J. M. (1995). How does cognitive therapy prevent depressive relapse and why should attentional control (mindfulness) training help? *Behaviour Research and Therapy, 33*(1), 25-29.

Telles, S., Hanumanthaiah, B., Nagarathna, R., & Nagendra, H. R. (1993). Improvement in static motor performance following yogic training of school children. *Perceptual and Motor Skills, 76*(3), 1264-1266.

Wood C., (1993). Mood change and perceptions of vitality: A comparison of the effects of relaxation, visualization and yoga. *Journal of the Royal Society of Medicine, 86*(5), 254-258.

Behavioral Health Plan

Acceptance Strategies

☐ I will make my lists of avoided psychological experiences and put them in a bowl on:

_____(when).

To help me move into a perspective of observing my thoughts during psychological acceptance practices, I will (check 2 or more):

☐ Use 4 deep breathes, counting each inhale.

☐ Use this visual image: _____.

☐ Use this verbal/auditory phrase:_____.

☐ I will practice the BOSE _____ (where) for _____.

minutes each day starting at _____ (time), beginning on _____ (date).

Strategies For Expressing Values

The area of life I will target for expressing my values is:

☐ Enjoying Things Alone   ☐ Sensual Experience

☐ Accomplishing Things Alone   ☐ Fun with Others

☐ Talking with Others   ☐ Images of a Better Future

☐ Contentment with Work

To improve my expression of values in this area, I will:

When:	Where:

With whom:

Who will support my plan?

As a reward for following my Behavioral Health Plan, I will:

Am I 100% committed to this Plan?   ☐ Yes   ☐ No

Chapter 3

Appreciating Your Mind and Body

Weekly Review

What parts of your Behavioral Health Plan did you complete during the past week? Were you able to generate a list of difficult psychological experiences? Did your mind wander during your practice periods? Did you notice arguments in your mind during practice? A pattern of conflict and argumentation is common in mental activity. Did you notice how quickly your mind slipped into dialogues of "is/is not" throughout the day. Are you remembering to count four deep breaths and gently bring yourself back to "observation level?" At "observation level," you see *more* of your life context and are more able to make choices that enhance your well-being. Take a moment now to use the goal attainment rating scales to assess your success in using acceptance strategies. Rate your ability to focus on your breath and your confidence in your ability "to give your mind a large, spacious meadow."

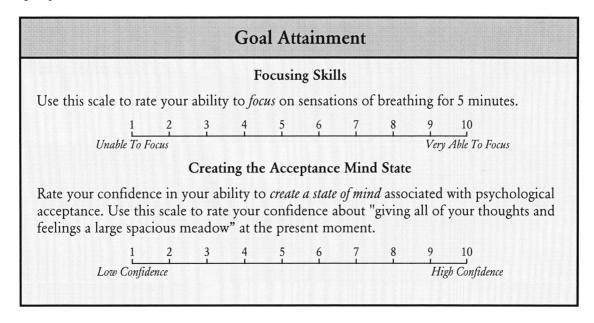

How do your ratings right now compare with your ratings in Chapter 2? Are your ratings this week lower or higher? Try moving to "observation level" at this very moment to watch any thoughts you are having about your present ratings. These skills are difficult to master. Continue to practice breath awareness and the process of being present with your experience. These are basic exercises for success in applying psychological acceptance strategies more consistently in your daily life. Skillfulness in this area will amplify results from application of other strategies suggested in this book. For example, accepting your mind and body paves the way to greater *appreciation* of your mind and body, which we will address in the present chapter.

Self-Assessment

Complete the method(s) of self-assessment that you choose to track your progress. You may photocopy the form(s) most useful to you from Appendix E. **If you are using the Quality of Life Scale** (QL Scale), compare your present ratings with your last ratings. How do they differ? Your feelings may become more intense when you begin to practice acceptance strategies. Over time, your ability to accept your feelings without a struggle will increase and, as this happens, the intensity of difficult feelings may lessen considerably. Are you using more coping strategies on a daily basis? Compare your ratings with last week's.

Did your Behavioral Health Plan have an impact on your ability to express your values in the area of life targeted by the plan? Often, a Behavioral Health Plan will enhance expression of values in the targeted area *and* several other areas. For example, Ben planned to call an old friend from his college days. He wanted to plan a fishing trip with his friend, who knew the local lakes well. In making this plan, Ben hoped to increase his satisfaction in "Talking with Others." While he had historically enjoyed a close circle of friends, he had stopped talking with his friends when his wife became terminally ill. Ben was his wife's primary care-giver and the sole bread winner in his family. His satisfaction ratings improved slightly in "Fun with Others" and "Accomplishments Alone," as he enjoyed reminiscing with his friend and he felt he handled his friend's questions about his deceased wife well.

What did you notice inside and outside of yourself while implementing your plan? Did you notice any uncomfortable sensations? Tension? Sadness? Self-critical thoughts? Self-doubting thoughts? Fearful images? When Ben dialed his friend's phone number, he noticed thoughts about getting tongue-tied, being a burden to his friend, and just wanting to be alone. He accepted these thoughts, breathed slowly with awareness, and spoke into the phone when his friend answered. He noticed warmth in his friend's voice and really enjoyed the laughter they shared when recalling a fishing trip of 15 years ago. After the call, Ben evaluated his experiment and decided to look for some old photographs of friends from college.

If you are using antidepressant medications, the Symptoms Checklist may help you identify specific symptom changes (See Appendix E). Monitoring your progress closely during the early weeks of therapy helps you notice small improvements. For example, Dan completed the Symptoms Checklist and noticed that he did not check concentration as a problem this week. This evidence of progress encouraged Dan to continue with the medication. Identification of the *early benefits* of antidepressant treatment is particularly important as troubling side effects are somewhat common during the first few weeks of treatment. Persevere and more medication benefits will develop over the next few weeks.

If you are using the Daily Wellness Check (DW Check), what were your highest and lowest daily ratings during the past week? How did these two days differ? What key thoughts or activities are associated with days when you "live life well?" Do you see themes or specific thoughts that recur in various situations? For example, Hannah noticed a tendency to ruminate about unpleasant moments of her day when she went to bed at night. She decided to practice acceptance strategies when she laid down to go to sleep. Over the week, she started to fall asleep more easily. Her DW Checks helped her see the extent to which improved sleep helped her "live life well." Take a moment to reflect and write down a few examples of thoughts and activities in your life that support the quality of life you want and deserve on a day-to-day basis. Use the "Discoveries" box.

Be prepared for change to develop gradually and with steps backwards, as well as forward. This is the nature of change. Continual assessment helps you see the bigger picture in behavioral change programs.

Discoveries from Daily Wellness Checks During the Past Week
1.
2.
3.
4.

Strategies: Appreciating Your Body and Mind

The goals of this chapter are to help you become more aware of your body and more able to create sensations of well-being in your body. The mind and body of the human being are miraculously complex and adaptable at any stage of life. In the first year of life, babies delight in raising their tiny hands to their mouths. During the second year, toddlers marvel at their ability to use their bodies to stand and walk. They spend many hours perfecting these complex abilities every day.

Unfortunately, as one grows older, one may forget how to observe and participate wholly and happily in the development of the vast range of abilities of mind and body. You may become more careful, more serious, more controlled, more indirect, more calculating. In short, you may become more "mental" in your approach to life. You may not feel the sensations of touch in a handshake. At times, you may feel as if you are a "head" moving through your day without a body attached. When was the last time you turned a cartwheel or clicked your heels together when you were excited? Do you allow yourself to laugh a "big belly" laugh when a humorous image comes into your mind? Do you hear leaves crunch when you step on them or see shapes in a cloudy sky? We can do these things and still be an adult. In fact, you will probably enjoy life more if you bring the body/mind abilities of childhood into your adult years.

Ashley Montagu, a British anthropologist, conducted a study of psychological neoteny (1992). Psychological neoteny refers to the presence of desirable childlike qualities in an adult. These qualities include spontaneity, generosity, uncontrollable laughter, curiosity, and open expression of feelings. Dr. Montagu notes that adults who are low in qualities of psychological neoteny can "re-learn" these activities. You were once highly aware of your mind and body. You still have the capacity to breathe full, natural breaths like an infant. With practice, your mind can help your body and your body can help your mind to live with more curiosity, spontaneity, laughter, trust, cooperation and joy.

Effectiveness: Body/Mind Strategies

Body/mind appreciation techniques are effective methods for improving numerous health problems, particularly problems related to tension. These techniques are helpful in preventing and treating substance abuse (Gelderloos, et al., 1991), particularly alcoholism (Taub, et al., 1994). Also, these skills help with mood management. Body/mind techniques also help people cope with stressful jobs. Managers have found these techniques helpful in creating greater job satisfaction (Heilbronn, 1992). Several Scandinavian researchers reported successful use of body/mind strategies to reduce anger (Dua & Swinden, 1992). Finally, selected body/mind strategies help people manage pain more effectively (Nespor, 1991). Kaplan (1993) reported that use of body/mind strategies for 10 weeks by 77 patients with fibromyalgia resulted in decreased pain.

Basic *body listening* skills may be helpful to patients with chronic illnesses (Price, 1993). Body/mind appreciation techniques have been determined to be an important part of prophylactic treatment for cancer and coronary heart disease (Grossarth-Maticek & Eysenck, 1991). Certain body/mind techniques improve brain functioning in patients with drug-resistant epilepsy (Deepak, et al., 1994). These techniques may help reduce frequency and intensity of headaches and lower blood pressure. Breathing retraining, in particular, helps reduce arousal and improve restorative workings within the body. Finally, according to Dr. Montagu, cultivation of neotenous qualities may result in hypertension improvement and living "longer *and* better."

Goal Setting

Before you start Skill Work on these powerful strategies, evaluate your present skill level and form goals. Use the two scales suggested in the Goal Setting box to evaluate (1) your ability to sustain concentration on bodily sensations and (2) your confidence in creating body/mind sensations of wellness. Try to increase your ratings in one (or both) of these areas, by one (or more) points during the coming week. Circle the number that indicates your skill level. Mark an "x" on the number corresponding to your goal.

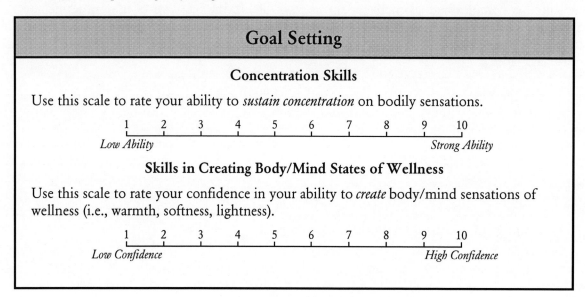

Skill Work: Body/Mind Awareness

Body and mind appreciation skills can be divided into two groups, which overlap considerably. The purpose of developing the first set of skills is to improve your ability to concentrate. Your work in practicing psychological acceptance will be useful to you here. The second group of skills helps you directly change your body/mind experience.

Awareness and Concentration Exercises

Experiment with the following three exercises. Choose the one that appeals to you. Daily practice helps maximize your benefit from these awareness-promoting exercises.

1. **Breathing Into The Body - 10 Areas.** Breathing techniques are useful tools for enhancing body awareness. Try this exercise while lying down or sitting in a chair or on the floor. Start by breathing deeply into your chest. Feel the sensations of your chest rising, as you take in air. Use words to label other sensations you notice. As you exhale, note the sensations of your chest falling as you let go of the air. Use a metaphor of "taking" and "letting go" to focus your attention as you explore sensations of breathing. Try breathing into specific areas of your body. Breathe into your stomach and explore the "taking in" sensations in your stomach. Breathe out and experience the sensations of "letting go" from your stomach. Continue with three *slow*, intentional breaths into each of the following ten areas of your body.

- Face
- Neck
- Shoulders
- Back
- Arms
- Hands
- Stomach
- Buttocks
- Legs
- Feet

In this awareness exercise, try to *follow rather than force* your breath. This procedure takes about 10 minutes. After several weeks of practice, you may be able to shorten the procedure, without loosing its impact, by reducing the number of breathes to each area or by *combining* areas of the body.

2. **Breathing Into the Body - 6 Areas.** A second breathing exercise is one suggested by Dr. James La Spira. You may do this exercise lying down or sitting in a chair or on the floor. In this exercise, you also focus on breathing into specific areas of the body. Your attention needs to be on the "sensations" of breathing into each of six areas of the body, one area at a time. All six areas in this exercise are in close proximity to the lungs. In each of the six areas, you count ten breaths, aloud or silently, noticing the sensations of the breath in the area of focus. The six areas form a circle around the chest area of your body, starting with the throat and ending with the shoulders. Practice taking ten breaths into each of the following six areas listed. After ten breaths to the throat area, move to the heart area for ten breaths, etc.

- Throat
- Middle, front of the lungs (heart area)
- Bottom, front of the lungs (diaphragm area)
- Bottom, back of the lungs (behind the diaphragm area)
- Middle, back of the lungs (behind the heart area)
- Top of the lungs (shoulder area)

When you lose count, start again at the beginning with the throat. With practice, you will be able to maintain your focus for ten breaths in each of the six areas. After you are able to attend to ten breaths in the six areas, add a second series of ten breaths in each area, starting with the shoulders and circling back to the throat.

3. **Tensing and Relaxing.** A second approach to increasing awareness of the body involves tensing each of the body parts listed above for the first breathing exercise (i.e., face, neck, shoulders, back, etc.). Tense each area separately for 5 to 7 seconds. Follow each 5- to 7-second period of tension with 20 to 30 seconds of relaxation. For each of the body areas, conduct two full cycles of tension and relaxation. If you have more difficulties in relaxing a particular area of your body, repeat the tension and relaxation cycle several additional times. This approach allows you to exaggerate the contrast between a tense and relaxed group of muscles. This method was developed by Dr. Edmond Jacobson in 1929. Use of an audio tape may help you develop proficiency more quickly. While you may purchase audio tapes instructing you in progressive relaxation, you often get the best results when you make your

own tape. Your own voice may deliver the message to you more effectively than a stranger's voice. If you have a lot of tension and are unable to make progress in using this exercise, consult a mental health provider with expertise in relaxation training. A professional can customize exercises to meet your particular needs. Relaxation is a very basic skill and very important to mental and physical health.

Skills for Influencing Body/Mind Experience

Both the breathing and the tensing-relaxing methods mentioned above have a positive influence on the mind and body. The muscles warm and become smooth. Your heart rate and blood pressure decrease. The following skills are imagery skills that can be used alone or combined with either the breathing or tensing-relaxing methods to help you obtain a deeper sense of well being.

1. **Using a Cue.** The use of an *imagined cue* prior to the start of practice of the breathing or tension-relaxation procedure is useful. The cue will become associated with heightened awareness of your body. Then, the cue alone can be used to prompt more body awareness during stressful moments. For example, Regan, a college student, used her personal cue, a turtle, to help her remember to slow down and check for tension prior to starting an exam or class presentation. Then, she gave her tense muscles a deep breath and said, "I am safe," silently to herself as she exhaled. She imagined the muscles warming and "smoothing out" under the protection of a resilient turtle shell. Then, like a turtle, she began a slow, intentional, graceful travel through the exam questions. Some people prefer to use a word or phrase *without* a visual image. Use your imagination to find the visual, auditory or multi-sensory image that will work for you.

2. **Using a Serenity Image.** A second imagery strategy involves painting a remembered or fantasized image of a serene environment for your own mind's eye. Practicing this image on a daily basis will help you learn to efficiently create the image and associated sensations of wellness during stressful moments of daily living.

3. **Aligning with Nature.** A third imagery technique is to align your body and mind with an element of nature that you find appealing. In *Wherever You Go, There You Are* (1994), Dr. Jon Kabat-Zinn suggested the use of a mountain or lake metaphor in mindfulness exercises. After repeatedly imaging your mind and body taking on the elements of a mountain, your mind and body may spontaneously experience the strength, diversity, receptivity, and serenity of the mountain during times of "bad weather." Jan, a busy family practice nurse, often felt tense by mid-morning. She began to practice the image of "rooting" herself in the ground, like a tree, during her 10:30 AM break. Jan developed a physical exercise to support her tree image. She stretched her spine toward the sky and extended her arms as it they were branches reaching for rays of sun. After reaching and breathing in the sun, she lowered her arms to the ground as if they were branches heavy with fruit. Jan practiced her exercise and image several times during her morning break. When she returned from break, she noticed that her neck and shoulders were more relaxed. She felt more receptive to the requests of her patients and co-workers. Her energy and optimism were better, and others noticed. Over time, Jan also experienced an increase in her physical strength and flexibility. Experiment with the image of becoming one with an image of a lake when you are laying on your bed. Imagine watching calmly and receptively, as a lake watches a bird flying or a leaf blowing over its surface. Imagine allowing a school of excited, hungry fish to move in one area while remaining a whole lake, deep and diverse in nature. When you have a night of interrupted sleep, work with this lake image. It is a restful image to use in caring for a worried and tired mind. Excellent tapes of the lake and mountain image are available from Dr. Kabat-Zinn.

4. **Cultivating Neoteny.** A fourth approach to increasing appreciation of your mind and body is to cultivate more neotenous qualities. If you are excessively serious, you may want to imagine engaging in childlike play activities. You will need to plan brief rollicking activities on a daily basis to strengthen this neotenous quality in your life, especially if your life circumstances run counter to your spending time frivolously. For example, Mike wanted to laugh more. He worked as an accountant in a large architecture firm. His colleagues were very serious. Mike began his neoteny program by observing others laugh. Then, he started to see comedy movies weekly. He bought a joke book and went to a comedy club several times. Eventually, his tendency to check his laughter faded and he developed a deep and vigorous laugh that generated more appreciation of himself and others.

Example: Body/Mind Strategies

Rich was a business man who thought little about his body or mind. He began to experience financial problems and noticed frequent headaches, blurred vision, and fatigue. His physician diagnosed high blood pressure, high cholesterol and diabetes. Rich felt disgusted with his body and demoralized by his life circumstances. His physician suggested a lifestyle consultation with the Behavioral Health Consultant in the clinic.

The consultant suggested some reading material, which Rich found interesting. As he learned more about the human body and reactions to stress, he became more interested in working creatively with his body. Rich practiced the breathing technique involving ten breaths to six areas encircling his chest. He also located an audio cassette series containing recordings of nature sounds. He took walks and listened to his tapes on a daily basis. As he walked, he focused on his breath. His headaches decreased, and he felt more optimistic about pursuing other lifestyle changes to control his diabetes. Rich began to explore poetry for the first time in his life. Additionally, he signed up for a community center class on photography.

Behavioral Health Plan: Applying Body/Mind Strategies

This week's plan asks you to select body/mind strategies for daily practice in the week ahead. Turn to the Behavioral Health Plan form at the end of this chapter and review it now. In the first section, indicate one or more strategies you plan to practice on a daily basis. Also, note the time and place you plan to practice any exercise(s) you indicate on the plan.

In the "Strategies for Expressing Your Values" section, select an area of your life that needs attention. A particularly good area for this week's plan is one where you lack awareness of your body *or* where you experience excessive tension. Choose an area that you believe you can improve through practice of body/mind appreciation or relaxation skills. Include use of an awareness or relaxation strategy in developing your plan to express what you value in this area. While "living life well" does not mean being free of tension, you may experience life with more joy when you are more aware and more calm.

As a part of your plan, do include receiving support from another person (a friend or a professional helper) if possible. Also, include a specific, planned small reward for yourself. Making planned changes is hard work. Acknowledge yourself for making the effort to create a better life.

Your commitment to the plan is essential. If you cannot commit 100% to your plan, revise it now. Often, when you enroll in a class to support your on-going practice of a method for developing more appreciation of your mind and body you obtain greater longer-term benefits. A list of classes that may support your development of strategies suggested in this chapter is located in Appendix F. Many of these classes may be available in community centers or other educational facilities in your neighborhood.

References

Deepak, K. K., Manchanda, S. K., & Maheshwari, M. C. (1994). Meditation improves clinicoelectroencephalographic measures in drug-resistant epileptics. *Biofeedback and Self Regulation, 19*(1), 25-40.

Dua, J. K., & Swinden, M. L. (1992). Effectiveness of negative-thought-reduction, meditation, and placebo training treatment in reducing anger. *Scandinavian Journal of Psychology, 33*(2), 135-146.

Gelderloos, P., Walton, K. G., Orme, J., David, W., & Alexander, C. N. (1991). Effectiveness of the transcendental meditation program in preventing and treating substance misuse: A review. *International Journal of the Addictions, 26*(3), 293-325.

Grossarth-Maticek, R., & Eysenck, H. J. (1991). Creative novation behaviour therapy as a prophylactic treatment for cancer and coronary heart disease: Part I description of treatment. *Behavior Research and Therapy, 29*(1), 1-16.

Heilbronn, F. S. (1992). The use of hatha yoga as a strategy for coping with stress in management development. *Management Education and Development, 23*(2), 131-139.

Jacobson, E. (1974). *Progressive relaxation.* Chicago: The University of Chicago Press, Midway Reprint.

Kabat-Zinn, J. (1994). *Wherever you go, there you are.* New York: Hyperion.

Kaplan, K. H. (1993). Goldenberg, D.L., Galvin, N.M. The impact of a meditation-based stress reduction program on fibromyalgia. *General Hospital Psychiatry, 15*(5), 294-299.

La Spira, J. (1995). Mindfulness workshop. *Society for Behavioral Medicine National Conference*, San Diego, CA.

Montagu, A. (1990). Psychological neoteny, *Longevity*, February.

Nespor, K. (1991). Pain management and yoga. *International Journal of Psychosomatics, (Special Issue) 38*(1-4), 76-91.

Price, M. J. (1993). Exploration of body listening: Health and physical self-awareness in chronic illness. *Advances in Nursing Science, 15*(4), 37-52.

Taub, E., Steiner, S. S., Weingarten, E., & Walton, K. G. (1994). Effectiveness of broad spectrum approaches to relapse prevention in severe alcoholism: A long-term, randomized, controlled trial of transcendental meditation, EMG biofeedback and electronic neurotherapy. Special Issue: Self-recovery: Treating addictions using transcendental meditation and maharishi ayurveda: I. *Alcoholism Treatment Quarterly, 11*(1-2), 187-220.

Behavioral Health Plan
Awareness And Body/Mind Integration Strategies

I will practice the following skills on a daily basis.

1. Awareness and Concentration Exercises:
   - ☐ Breathing Into the Body: ☐ 10 Areas or ☐ 6 Areas
   - ☐ Tensing and Relaxing

2. Exercises to Increase Body/Mind Integration:
   - ☐ Using A Cue
   - ☐ Using A Serenity Image
   - ☐ Aligning with Nature
   - ☐ Cultivating Neoteny through Planned Behavioral Activities, including:

Strategies For Expressing Values

The area of life I will target for expressing my values is:

☐ Enjoying Things Alone	☐ Sensual Experience
☐ Accomplishing Things Alone	☐ Fun with Others
☐ Talking with Others	☐ Images of a Better Future
☐ Contentment with Work	

To enhance my expression of values in this area, I will:

When:	Where:

With whom:

Who will support my plan?

As a reward for following my Behavioral Health Plan, I will:

Am I 100% committed to this Plan?   ☐ Yes   ☐ No

Chapter 4

Solving Problems

Weekly Review

Last week, you began experimenting with exercises to enhance your ability to use body/mind techniques to improve your quality of life. What parts of your Behavioral Health Plan did you complete? What did you notice about physical sensations of tension and relaxation, and your ability to *create* sensations of wellness? Take a moment now to evaluate your skills in these important areas. Use the scales in the Goal Attainment box to indicate your ability to sustain concentration on bodily sensations and your ability to create body/mind sensations of wellness.

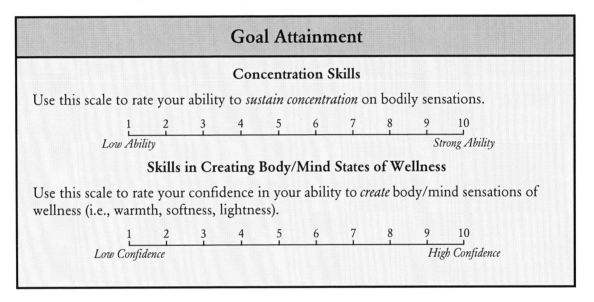

Compare your ratings with the ratings you made in the Goal Setting box in Chapter 3. Have your ratings improved, even slightly? Continued practice of exercises in Chapter 3 will help you strengthen skills in this area. Progressive relaxation techniques may be mastered in several weeks. However, the totality of benefit from systematic relaxation procedures and other body/mind techniques requires months and even years of on-going practice.

If you are struggling with implementation of your Behavioral Health Plans, this chapter may help you identify and address obstacles. This chapter offers you an opportunity to review problem-solving skills and apply them to an area of life that is challenging for you right now. Remember to acknowledge your "mini-successes" in working toward wellness. Even when your behavioral health plan does not unfold as planned, you learn from the results when you take the time to reflect and review. Pay attention and *let your experience be your teacher*.

Self-Assessment

Complete the method(s) of self-assessment that you chose to track your progress. You may photocopy the form(s) most useful to you from Appendix E. **If you are using the Quality of Life Scale (QL Scale), compare this week's ratings with those from last week. Do they differ? Using** exercises suggested in Chapter 3 may influence your QL ratings in several ways. First, exercises designed to increase your awareness probably increased your attention to the sensations associated with emotional experience. You may have noticed that your chest tightens when you are angry or your eyes sting when you are sad. Did your feelings seem more intense? Did you use more coping strategies? An increased "sense of calm" may have a pervasive effect on quality of life.

Did your Behavioral Health Plan have an impact on your value-expression ratings in the area targeted by the plan? Mrs. Johnson planned to improve her satisfaction in the area of "Accomplishing Things Alone." She struggled with assuming new responsibilities after the death of her husband of forty-eight years. Paying bills was a disquieting task that required weekly attention. Mrs. Johnson's neck often ached after paying bills. She occasionally experienced a headache. Mrs. Johnson valued her independence. She wanted to continue to pay her own bills and to do so with more confidence and a sense of calm. She reasoned that she would feel more calm and confident during bill-paying sessions if she were more relaxed. She developed an image of serenity–a scene from her childhood on a farm. She practiced a cue ("Life is good.") just prior to practicing her serenity image. With daily practice, the cue began to provoke relaxation by itself. After 6 days of practice, Mrs. Johnson used her cue before sitting down to pay bills. She checked her shoulders before she started working. Whenever she noticed tension in her shoulders, she stopped to repeat her cue and take a slow, deep breath. She had no neck or shoulder pain when she completed her finance work, and she noticed a significant increase in her ratings concerning expression of values (i.e., confidence, calmness, independence) in the category of "Accomplishing Things Alone."

Jeff, a computer programmer who worked long hours, obtained desired results from his Behavioral Health Plan. He planned to target "Sensual Experience" and found that his ratings on "Images of a Better Future" and "Fun Activities Alone" increased as well. Jeff's Behavioral Health Plan included daily practice of one of the breathing techniques suggested in Chapter 3 and experimentation with psychological neoteny. He decided to visit a local bakery with a "childlike" frame of mind. At the bakery, he "smelled" wonderful things, selected a big peanut butter cookie, and whistled a favorite tune on his way to a table in the bakery. All of these "neotenous" behaviors were quite different from Jeff's usual serious approach to life. While he felt awkward, he liked the tingle of "playfulness" he perceived in his body. Did your ratings of satisfaction with life change in ways you predicted?

If you are using antidepressant medications, the Symptoms Checklist may help you identify specific symptom changes (See Appendix E). Monitoring your progress closely during the early weeks of therapy helps you detect small improvements. For example, Emily completed the Symptoms Checklist and noticed that she did not check sadness as a problem this week. Upon reflection, she realized how subtle this change in mood had been. This evidence of progress encouraged her to continue with medication. Identification of the *early benefits* of antidepressant treatment is particularly important when you have reservations about use of medications. Emily had felt she should not "have to use medications to manage her life." She now realized that her behavioral work was as important, if not more important, than her use of medications. She saw that use of an antidepressant probably helped her implement initial behavioral plans. Emily also felt some satisfaction in knowing that her continued use of behavioral strategies would help prevent her future need for use of medications.

If you are using the Daily Wellness Check (DW Check), what were your highest and lowest daily ratings during the past week? How did these two days differ? What key thoughts or activities are associated with your days when you "live life well?" Do you see some themes that recur in various situations? For example, Dick noticed a tendency to spend much of his afternoon walk reviewing difficult moments he had at work that day. When Dick decided to spend the first five minutes of his walk attending to his environment, his breathing ("taking in" and "letting go") and his body, he found that he ended the walk with a deeper sense of relaxation. His daily ratings were higher, reflecting a greater sense of "living life well" associated with this small change. Take a moment to reflect on your daily ratings. Write down any thoughts and activities in your life that provide you with higher quality experiences. These observations may help you "fine tune" behavioral health plans.

Discoveries from Daily Wellness Checks During the Past Week
1.
2.
3.
4.

Strategies: Building Self-Efficacy and Problem-Solving Skills

Dr. Albert Bandura suggests that "self-efficacy" is an important part of living life well. Self-efficacy is your belief in your ability to cope with what life brings you. It is your confidence in being able to "put it on the line" when the time comes. When your self-efficacy about a situation is high, your response to that situation is likely to be effective. In fact, Dr. Bandura has demonstrated that high self-efficacy predicts success when a person attempts to address new or very difficult stresses and to make lifestyle changes that accommodate problems.

Self-efficacy is a reflection of your confidence in solving specific problems as you encounter them. Mastery of problem-solving skills improves your confidence and, hence, your self-efficacy Research findings suggest that people believe they can solve problems when they are able to identify specific coping strategies and apply them with confidence (Larson, et al., 1990). The most effective strategies are those that represent a stance of *positive action*. Positive problem-solving strategies include embracing difficult psychological experiences, increasing sensations of wellness in the body, and systematically applying problem-solving steps to unresolved stresses.

Strategies in this chapter help you increase your self-efficacy, or confidence, *and* skills in addressing unresolved problems in your life. At present, you may be using less active or avoidant approaches to problems you do not know how to solve. The most difficult step in transforming a passive, avoidant problem-solving strategy into a positive one is "*taking the first step*." The first step is usually that of *identifying that something is a problem*. Lazarus identifies other early steps in solving difficult problems. These include: accepting the possibility that something can be done about a problem, expressing a desire to change, and being willing to work and to make an effort to change.

You may find yourself "stuck" at step one, with your head in the sand like an ostrich. The problems in our lives that limit us most are those that are unrecognized. Investigate problems you tend to deny or minimize. Are you using a negative problem-solving strategy to address a difficult problem? What are the costs and benefits of continuing to use this strategy? Personal change begins with acceptance of the problem as a problem that can be addressed more effectively.

In the book, *Nothing Special* (1993), Beck and Smith tell an old Sufi story about a person who dropped his keys on the dark side of the street at night. He crossed the street to be near the lamppost. On the light side of the street, he began to look for his keys. His friend witnessed the whole scene. The friend went to the person and asked why he was looking under the lamp instead of where he dropped his keys. He replied, "I am looking here because there is more light." You may find yourself doing this at times–applying a problem-solving strategy that is clearly off the mark.

While problems may be very complex, all have solutions. However, the solution may not relate *directly* to the problem. For example, engaging in regular exercise or relaxation activities reduces heavy use of mind-altering substances, such as alcohol or marijuana. While the solution of exercising is not directly related to the substance abuse, it may have a profound effect upon the problem of substance abuse.

We are also hesitant to see a problem as a problem if we anticipate that the solution to the problem will result in other problems. For example, Louise lost her job. She saw herself as reliant on her critical husband for support. While she was dissatisfied with her marriage, she failed to take positive action to address marital problems. She adopted a "Don't rock the boat" philosophy. This negative problem-solving strategy conflicted with Louise's belief that she could create a loving and satisfying relationship with another person. To some extent, Louise reconciled this value conflict by blaming herself for failing to obtain approval from her husband and failing to create the loving relationship she wanted. She felt discouraged. She was "stuck" and needed to use active problem-solving efforts to improve her life.

When we find ourselves depending on another person, we need to question the necessity of this orientation in the relationship. Perceiving yourself as dependent on another may conflict with engaging in autonomous problem-solving behavior. This is particularly true when we associate our welfare with the other person's acceptance of us. Unfortunately, the intimacy we seek in such a relationship eludes us. Instead of closeness, we find frustration. After seeing a counselor, Louise began to use more active problem-solving strategies to solve her dilemma. One of her first steps was to pursue an autonomous solution. She took a part-time job outside of her field in order to provide some income for her family and to expose herself to social interactions outside the troubled marriage.

Autonomy underlies self-efficacy. Questioning your dependencies is an important part of living life well. Are your dependencies in keeping with your values? Dr. William Glasser suggests use of *positive addictions* to solve problems posed by unworkable dependencies or habits. A positive addiction is an activity that is non-competitive, can be done daily in an hour or less, is easy to do alone (and does not depend on others), is believed to be of mental, spiritual, or physical value (and is "measured" by you alone), and can be done without criticism from yourself or others. These types of activities are often viable solutions to unwanted and unchangeable circumstances in life. Examples of positive addictions include jogging, listening to opera, watching birds or other animals, and working crossword puzzles.

Finally, the overlooked obstacle to solving a difficult problem may be that you are not identifying resources that are potentially available to you. Identifying overlooked resources may involve believing that a solution is possible. Remembering past successes in solving similar difficulties may help. Unfortunately, *memory is mood dependent.* This means that you tend to remember experiences that "fit" your mood of the moment. If you are discouraged, you may focus more on past experiences where you were lacking in self-efficacy. Your mood will change, even if you do nothing to change it, because life will offer up something and you will respond. If you want to shift your mood *intentionally*, you can do so by engaging in an enjoyable activity or recollecting a time when you felt better. When your mood is more positive, you can more easily recall the specifics of past successes you have had in coping with adverse circumstances that are similar to present life problems.

Effective problem-solving leads to development of goals. Of course, you will need to decide which goals and which steps come first. In a sense, there is no such thing as a wrong solution because all of your efforts will give you information to use in planing your next move. It was a wise person who said, "Mistakes are a good way to learn." When living life well, you form goals and work toward them, while being aware of and learning from your moment-to-moment experience, including mistakes.

Effectiveness: Problem-Solving

Use of effective problem-solving strategies is associated with mental and physical wellness. Individuals who respond to major negative life change with more problem-focused coping responses display fewer signs of depression (Billings & Moos, 1981). More effective problem-solvers consistently report fewer signs of depression than less effective problem-solvers (Nezu, 1985; Nezu, et al., 1986). Nezu studied people who had suffered a diverse array of life stresses and were demoralized or depressed. He found that people who attended problem-focused group sessions or classes reported significantly more improvements in mood, problem-solving skills, and a greater sense of internal direction than people who did not attend the sessions.

Kim-Berg and DeShazer (1986) reported that people who focus on solutions are likely to attain goals related to solving many different kinds of life problems and to be very satisfied with brief use of counseling experts. An English psychiatrist taught primary care physicians to support their patients in using problem-solving skills (Mynors-Wallace & Gath, 1995). He found that patients who received support from their physician in using problem-solving skills reported more improvement in mood and more optimism about their future than patients who did not receive this support. Rehm, Kaslow, and Rabin (1987) reported promising results from a self-control program, which involved use of problem-solving. Finally, use of problem-solving strategies helps couples resolve marital conflicts and improve marital satisfaction (Jacobson & Gurman, 1986).

In fact, self-efficacy may be the core of living life well. Self-efficacy is an attitude of "I can do it, I am in charge of how I conduct my life." Rodin and Langer (1992) found that nursing home residents who were encouraged to *make decisions* for themselves (e.g., about where they visited with guests) and to *take responsibility* for caring for a plant died at half the rate of patients who were encouraged to let staff members make decisions for them and take care of plants for them. Responsibly solving problems is very important to *staying alive* as well as living well.

Goal Setting

Use the scales in the Goal Setting box to estimate your present level of self-efficacy and actual problem-solving skills concerning a specific problem in a specific area of your life. For example, you might select "Contentment with Work" as a focus and define the problem as "making more money." Alternatively, you might target "Accomplishing Things Alone" and define the problem as "taking better care of my yard." Choose an area of life to target and a problem focus in that area and circle the number that represents your confidence or ability now. Mark an "x" on the number you designate as your goal. You will apply powerful strategies to this problem and evaluate your progress in the Goal Attainment box in Chapter 5.

Skill Work: Problem-Solving

Apply the following steps to the problem you have selected for your Behavioral Health Plan. Because you are selecting a difficult problem, you will need to attend closely to the skill work exercises. You may want to review your work with a friend. The seven steps of problem-solving are powerful and require that you follow them with exactness (Nazu, 1985; Gath, 1990).

Step One: Pinpoint the Problem.

Further define the problem area. Describe the problem in several sentences. Remember that using psychological acceptance can help you avoid the trap of "being right" or becoming stuck on the issue of "fairness." Body/mind awareness will help you detect and short circuit "negative energy" associated with this problem.

Goal Setting

Decide on one of the seven areas of life to target in your Behavioral Health Plan. Within that area of your life, choose a specific problem. Make your ratings in regards to this selected problem.

Self Efficacy

Concerning your selected problem, rate your *confidence* (or self-efficacy) in your ability to make progress in solving this problem.

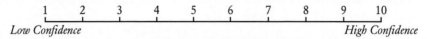

Low Confidence   *High Confidence*

Problem-Solving Skills

Concerning your selected problem, rate your abilities for implementing the first few steps in solving this problem.

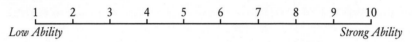

Low Ability   *Strong Ability*

For example, Gina chose to stop working and stay home when her young daughter was born. After several years of full-time mothering, she began to miss working outside of the home. Prior to the birth of her daughter, she had worked as a graphic artist and enjoyed her work. Whenever she allowed herself to explore returning to employment outside of the home, she was flooded with thoughts about "letting her daughter down" and "not being a good mother." While she was becoming increasingly uncomfortable with being at home full-time, she was stuck there given her unwillingness to experience her guilt and think through her options. Her efforts to pinpoint a problem in the area of "Contentment with Work" led to the following **descriptions of the problem**.

Problem Descriptions

1. I am uncomfortable with my thoughts about "letting my daughter down" and "not being a good mother."

1. I am isolated from working mothers and do not know if they experience these thoughts when they return to work or how they cope with them if they do.

1. I am afraid that my husband will be disappointed if I want to leave our daughter in a daycare situation.

Step Two: Brainstorm Solutions.

Ask yourself the following questions: "What would be different if this was less of a problem for me?" When Gina asked herself this, she generated the following **possible solutions**.

Possible Solutions
1. I would balance my thoughts by reminding myself that I am a good mother.
1. I would call one of my old friends who has two children, is divorced, and works full-time.
1. I would ask my husband what he thinks about my working part-time.
1. I would visit several home daycare situations alone and with my daughter to see how each of us respond.

Step Three: Evaluate Potential Solutions.

This requires that you *match your present resources with the potential action steps that you could take* to solve the problem. Gina did not feel that she could be successful in "balancing" her thoughts, and she was reluctant to call her friend who was a divorced, working mother. She was willing to talk with her husband, but felt he would be reluctant to support her return to work outside the home without knowing more about day care options. She chose to implement the alternative of exploring day care possibilities for her daughter.

Step Four: Identify Your First Step(s).

This requires that you commit to one or more specific, small action steps. After making a list of your first action step or steps, ask yourself, "If I do this, does it mean that I am making progress toward my goal?" Gina planned the following **steps for the first week** of her problem-solving program.

Day of the Week	Action Step
Monday	Form a list of questions to use to evaluate a potential day care placement
Tuesday	Call a day care referral service
Wednesday	Call to arrange several visits to centers
Thursday	Visit one or more centers
Friday	Take my daughter for a visit to the center I like best
Saturday	Discuss the results of problem-solving efforts with my husband

Step Five: Imagine success and anticipate obstacles.

Imagine success, and *anticipate and prepare for obstacles*. Gina anticipated that getting a baby-sitter for her daughter on Thursday might be an obstacle for her, so she planned to call her husband's aunt and ask her to watch her daughter. Gina feared that the aunt might ask where she planned to go. Gina did not want to reveal this, as she felt unsure of her direction at the present. Gina decided that she would tell the aunt she planned to "run errands." Further, she decided that she would only reiterate this explanation if the aunt inquired again when she left her daughter at the aunt's apartment.

Step Six: Do It . . . Follow The Plan.

Follow the plan when the time comes. Gina checked off each of her action steps as she did them. She carefully observed her own reactions to each step.

Step Seven: Evaluate the Results and Continue Planning.

Pretend that you are a scientist. Look at your results objectively. Continue working toward the solution or goal by simply determining and planning a next step or by going through these seven steps again. Gina found a home center operated by a grandmotherly woman in her neighborhood. When she took her daughter for a visit, the daughter played with toys and talked with the woman comfortably. Later, she talked with her husband, and he indicated an interest in visiting the home-care center during the following week. Gina planned additional problem-solving steps, including placing her daughter in the home-care program one morning each week. She made a list of job search activities that she would pursue on the morning when her daughter was in the home-care program.

Skill Work: Problem-Solving Worksheet

Use the Problem-Solving Worksheet to develop an initial plan on the problem you want to target in the coming week. You may want to discuss your work with your "helper" or support person.

Example: Problem-Solving

Ricardo worked long hours at his job as a machinist. He took pride in his ability to support his wife and their children. When he was not at work, he spent most of his time working on his home or being with his wife and children. He missed having time alone and, in particular, he longed for time to play his guitar. Ricardo had once played in a band, and he missed seeing his musician friends. Ricardo believed that playing the guitar would be a relaxing and enjoyable activity for him and would add meaning to his life. Ricardo chose to use problem-solving skills concerning the area of "Fun Activities Alone" and to pinpoint the problem of having no time alone to play his guitar. His brainstorming produced the following potential solutions:

Possible Solutions
1. **Ask my wife to take the children away from the house for an hour on Sunday afternoon so that I can play guitar alone then.**
2. **Take my guitar to work and play for a half-hour during lunch.**
3. **Get up a half-hour earlier several mornings each week to play my guitar.**

Ricardo evaluated the potential solutions and decided not to ask his wife to take the children away for an hour on Sundays. His wife spent a great deal of her time caring for the children and needed alone time herself. He did not believe that he would get up earlier to play because he usually needed to sleep in order to feel rested and ready for the day. Ricardo chose to go with the idea of taking his guitar to work and playing during his lunch hour.

Problem-Solving Worksheet

Step One: Pinpoint the Problem.

Choose one of the following areas of your life to target in your problem-solving plan.

☐ *Enjoying Things Alone*   ☐ *Sensual Experience*

☐ *Accomplishing Things Alone*   ☐ *Fun with Others*

☐ *Talking with Others*   ☐ *Images of a Better Future*

☐ *Contentment with Work*

Describe a problem within the selected area. Define 3 or 4 aspects of the problem.

1.

2.

3.

4.

Step Two: Brainstorm solutions. Ask yourself the following questions: "What would be different if this was less of a problem for me?"

List several possible solutions.

1.

2.

3.

4.

Step Three: Evaluate potential solutions. This requires that you *match your present resources with the potential action steps that you might* take to solve the problem.

Solution Action Steps	Available Resources
1.	1.
2.	2.
3.	3.

Step Four: Identify your first step(s). This requires that you commit to one or more specific, small action steps. After making a list of your first action step or steps, ask yourself, "If I do this, does it mean that I am making progress toward my goal?"

Day of the Week	Action Step

Step Five: Imagine success and anticipate obstacles. *Make specific plans to address obstacles you may encounter.*

Action Step	Anticipated Obstacle	Plan to Address Obstacle

Step Six: Do it–follow the plan. Proceed with the plan when the time comes.

When:	Where:

With Whom:

Step Seven: Evaluate the Results and Continue Planning. Pretend that you are a scientist. Look at your results objectively. Continue working toward the solution or goal by simply determining and planning a next step or by going through these seven steps again.

Anticipated Result	Actual Result	Discrepancy

Next step(s):

Example

Ricardo developed the following action steps.

Day of the Week	Action Step
Saturday	Get new strings for guitar
Sunday	Put guitar and strings in truck
Monday	String and tune guitar at lunch
Tuesday	Play guitar for a half-hour during lunch break
Wednesday	Play guitar for a half-hour during lunch break
Thursday	Play guitar for a half-hour during lunch break
Friday	Play guitar for a half-hour during lunch break

He realized that finding a quiet place where he would not be interrupted could be a problem and planned for this potential obstacle. He spoke with his boss, who agreed to let him play in a storage room that was rarely used by anyone during lunch hour. Ricardo implemented his plan and attended to his experiences as he did so. He was surprised at how long it took him to string his guitar and at how slowly his facility in playing chords returned. He planned to continue his practice as it did provide more satisfaction with "Enjoying Things Alone" *and* "Accomplishing Things Alone."

Behavioral Health Plan: Problem-Solving Strategies

This chapter's Behavioral Health Plan requires you to identify a problem and complete a Problem-Solving Worksheet. You have already completed a great deal of the work by responding to Skill Work exercises. Complete the first section of your plan now. Additionally, identify who (or what) might be a resource for you in solving this problem. Resource identification is very important on this plan because you are tackling a particularly difficult problem. Having multiple resources for support will help your self-efficacy. Finally, set up a date for evaluating the results of your first problem-solving plan concerning this challenging circumstance.

In the section concerning expression of your values, indicate the area of life you plan to target. Identify one or more action steps you plan to take to address the selected problem. State the specifics of when, where, etc. Remember to identify your "helper" and your reinforcer. Check your commitment level. If it is not high, reconsider your plan. Does it require you to take too big of a step? Do you need more support to implement the plan? Find a way to improve your confidence in and commitment to the plan. If you feel "stuck," re-read this chapter and consider consulting with a psychologist or counselor. You may need the assistance of an expert in solving some problems.

References

Bandura, A. (1977). *Social learning theory*. Englewood Cliffs, N.J.: Prentice Hall.

Beck, C. H., & Smith, S. (1993). *Nothing special: Living Zen*. New York, N.Y.: Harper Collins Publishers.

Billings, A. G., & Moos, R. H. (1981). The role of coping responses and social resources in attenuating the stress of life events. *Journal of Behavioral Medicine, 4,* 139-17.

deShazer, S., Kim-Berg, I., Lipchik, E., Nunnally, E., Molnar, A., Gingrich, W., & Weiner-Davis, M. (1986). Brief therapy: Focused solution development. *Family Process, 25,* 207-221.

Jacobson, N. S., & Gurman, A. S. (1986). *Clinical handbook of marital therapy*. New York: Guilford.

Gath, D. *Problem solving therapy: A manual for primary care treatment of depression*, Unpublished.

Glaser, W. (1976). *Positive Addictions*. New York: Harper & Row.

Larson, L., Piersel, W. C., Imao, R. A., & Allen, S. J. (1990). Significant predictors of problem-solving appraisal. *Journal of Counseling Psychology, 37*(4), 482-490.

Mynors-Wallace, L., Gath, D. H., Lloyd-Thomas, A.R., & Tomlinson, D. (1995). Randomized controlled trial comparing problem-solving treatment with amitriptyline and placebo for major depression in primary care. *British Medical Journal, 310,* 441-446.

Nezu, A. M. (1985). Differences in psychological distress between effective and ineffective problem solvers. *Journal of Counseling Psychology, 32,* 135-138.

Nezu, A. M. (1986). Efficacy of a social problem-solving therapy approach for unipolar depression. *Journal of Consulting and Clinical Psychology, 54,* 196-202.

Nezu, A. M., Nezu, C.M., & Perri, M.G. (1989). *Problem solving therapy for depression*. New York: John Wiley & Sons.

Rehm, L. P., Kaslow, N. J., & Rabin, A. S. (1987). Cognitive and behavioral targets in a self-control therapy program. *Journal of Consulting and Clinical Psychology, 55,* 60-67.

Rodin, J., & Langer, E. See Langer, E. J. (1992). Matters of mind: Mindfulness/mindlessness in perspective. *Consciousness and Cognition: An International Journal, 1*(4), 289-305.

Behavioral Health Plan
Problem-Solving Strategies
I will focus on a new solution to the following problem this week:
I will complete a Problem-Solving Worksheet on: (date).
Who is a resource for me in solving this problem?
I will evaluate my results: (date).
Strategies For Expressing Values
The area of life I will target for expressing my values is:

☐ *Enjoying Things Alone*   ☐ *Sensual Experience*

☐ *Accomplishing Things Alone*   ☐ *Fun with Others*

☐ *Talking with Others*   ☐ *Images of a Better Future*

☐ *Contentment with Work*

To improve my expression of values in this area, I will:

When:	Where:
With whom:	
Who will support my plan?	
As a reward for following my Behavioral Health Plan, I will:	
Am I 100% committed to this Plan? ☐ Yes ☐ No	

Chapter 5

Responding To Interpersonal Conflicts

Weekly Review

Last week you started a process of systematically applying specific problem-solving skills to an area of life where you feel dissatisfied and discouraged. I hope that you implemented your "first steps" and that you are now ready to plan where to "plant your feet" for the next move in creating a better life. Take a moment now to evaluate your confidence in using formal problem-solving skills. Use the scaling questions in the Goal Attainment box to rate your confidence and abilities at the present moment. Compare your present ratings with your ratings in the Goal Setting box in Chapter 4. Continue to identify and use potential supportive resources for positive problem-solving both inside yourself and outside yourself. Resources create pathways for continued work on difficult problems.

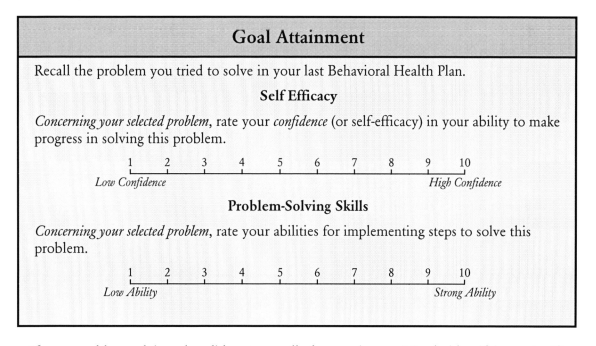

If your problem solving plan did not go well, do not give up. Merely identifying a significant problem is an accomplishment. Your next step in solving a difficult problem might be consulting a behavioral health specialist. She/he may help in several ways, including helping you redefine the problem or discover new potential solutions.

In this Chapter, you will learn more about knowing and caring for yourself in interpersonal conflict situations–which are replete with troublesome moments for most of us. These exercises may enhance your potential for success in using the problem-solving skills suggested in Chapter 4. In this chapter, you learn about specific procedures for *resolving uncertainties with others*. These methods work best when applied with a great deal of self-awareness. Effective problem-solving and high self-efficacy are hallmarks of a life lived well. Continue to practice these skills.

Self-Assessment

Complete the method(s) of self-assessment that you chose to track your progress. You may photocopy the form(s) most useful to you from Appendix E. **If you are using the Quality of Life Scale** (QL Scale), compare your Emotional Experience and Behavioral Action ratings for this week with those from last week. Do they differ? Using exercises from Chapter 4 may result in improved ratings in both areas. Additionally, effective problem-solving usually has a positive impact on your ability to demonstrate your values in many areas of living. Take a moment to total your scores on demonstrating your values in the seven areas of life. Compare this total with the total from your ratings in Chapter 4.

Reflect on your Behavioral Health Plan. What problem-solving steps were easier for you? Which were more difficult? Were you able to use acceptance and body/mind strategies to help you embrace negative thoughts about self *and* enter difficult situations with a greater sense of calm?

Angelica targeted "Talking with Others." Her plan involved discussion of a sensitive issue with her mother. She struggled with brain-storming possible solutions to propose to her mother. When she could only generate two solutions, she decided to consult a counselor at the student health clinic. The counselor asked questions to help her discover new solutions for further consideration. She decided to propose a solution that she discovered in her brainstorming session with the counselor. Her mother was impressed by her daughter's thoughtful presentation and the discussion went well.

If you are using medications, the Symptoms Checklist may be useful to you in evaluating the completeness of your response to antidepressant medications (See Appendix E). If sleep has been problematic for you, you are probably noticing significant improvement at this point in treatment. Marie found that she started to sleep better in her fourth week of antidepressant treatment. During the first few weeks, she had noted improved concentration and energy. Also, she felt more calm. If you are using medications and are still experiencing numerous symptoms on the checklist, do visit your doctor soon. Take the results of your checklist evaluation with you.

If you are using the Daily Wellness Check (DW Check), what were your highest and lowest daily ratings during the past week? How did these two days differ? What key thoughts or activities are associated with days when you "live life well?" Do you see patterns in your thinking or behavior that support effective problem solving? Lynn, a working mother, discovered a theme related to "choosing the easy way." Her daily ratings were higher on days *when her solutions to problems eased the burden of work on her*. For example, Monday was a better day because she bought brownies for her daughter's book club rather than trying to make them before she went to her office. Thursday was a better day because she changed the dinner plan from homemade pizza to soup and make-your-own sandwich. Lynn noted the following thoughts as supporting her solutions.

Lynn's Discoveries from Daily Wellness Checks During the Past Week
1. "This is good enough."
2. "I don't need to be super-Mom."

Take a moment to reflect on your daily ratings for the past week. Write down thoughts and activities in your life that are associated with a higher quality of life. Note any observations that may help with developing future behavioral health plans.

Even if change in your assessment ratings is minimal or lacking, *learn from what you did. There are no wrong plans or decisions*–only results that can provide valuable information. Take time to review and reflect upon your experiences when plans do not yield predicted results. Mistakes are a great way to learn.

If you have not yet tried the Daily Wellness Check method, consider trying it this week. It is particularly useful as an adjunct to the strategies and skills suggested in Chapters 5 and 6. Further, **the Daily Wellness Check can be turned into a positive habit of "daily review" after you "graduate"** from your work in this book.

Discoveries from Daily Wellness Checks During the Past Week
1.
2.
3.
4.

Strategies: Solving Interpersonal Problems

The only way to avoid *conflict* with other human beings is to avoid *contact* with other human beings. When we avoid others, we tend to feel "out of touch" with ourselves as well as others. Touch is an important strategy for communicating with others. Montagu identifies touch as central to physical and psychological well-being. In conflict situations, we often avoid or prohibit touch. Affiliating, caring and touching are a central part of being human. We prefer to be with others, to touch, and to communicate well.

Conflict is the price we must pay to "connect" with others. Strategies for working effectively with conflict will help you express your values, solve problems effectively and communicate effectively. These strategies are difficult to master. For example, most of us have difficulties accepting our initial feelings in a conflict situation. When we are unable to embrace or at least acknowledge these feelings, we tend to "turn them off" by taking action to avoid, increase, or stop the conflict. We defend ourselves or blame the other person. We excuse ourselves from the situation or "blow it up."

Whether you argue with your employer or your spouse, the human tendency is to see the other person as the problem. We often use language in these difficult moments to exacerbate anger, sadness, and pain. You may find yourself saying things, such as: "She only wants to hurt me," "He doesn't value my work," "I'll get even with them." These sentences lead us into painful *mind trips* and even more painful avoidance strategies. At these moments, applying psychological acceptance and self-awareness strategies is very difficult *and* very necessary in order to resolve conflicts effectively.

Certain patterns of responding to conflict may cost more than you want to pay. If we believe we must avoid conflict, we may withhold information needed to create healthy, growing relationships. We may sacrifice self respect in order to maintain the status quo. We may passively punish a person for a remark perceived as offensive by withdrawing from that person. On the other hand, we may seek power and control over another more directly. We may use our language and body to frighten others. When this is the case, one suffers from experience of excessive anger. High levels of anger appear to increase one's vulnerability to heart disease. Further, angry people are likely to have few, if any, friends.

Your "triggers" for conflict are created by your prior life experiences. Take a moment to review the "Be Right" and "It's Not Fair" agendas presented in Chapter 2, as they are common in interpersonal conflicts. Both leave us feeling cheated and alone. There is no need to invite, encourage, exacerbate, or cling to these feelings when your goal is to live life well.

Even in our darkest moments, we live in a world where interdependence is the rule. Addressing conflicts from the "big picture" perspective of interdependence can lead to different solutions. This is true whether the conflict is between you and your neighbor or the United States and another country. When you see the conflict in the larger context, you are more able to free yourself from the constrictive "literality" of "words" in the argument. In his book, *Putting Difference to Work*, Dr. Steve deShazer (1991) describes conflicts as occurring within "language games." He explains:

> The signs (or moves) during the game consist of sentences (or signs), which are made up of words, gestures, facial expressions, postures, thoughts, etc. Since this is a system complete in itself, any particular sign can only be understood within the context of the pattern of the activities involved. Thus, the meaning of any one word depends entirely on how the participants in the language game use that word. If the context were significantly different, that game would not be played; it would be a different game altogether (p. 73).

You have the power to change the system of conflict by changing yourself. A system changes significantly when one person changes his or her functioning within the system ever so slightly. Joko Beck (1993) explains that we can walk out on relationships, but we cannot leave them, as we remain in the system of conflict. Similarly, diplomats can walk out on peace talks but they cannot leave the world. Your experience of others in the conflict system continues inside of you. The social current tells us to "look out for number one" and, if we swim with this current, we see others as "out to get us." All benefit when you change your initial assumption about conflict. A position of responsible trust in yourself and the world empowers you to solve conflicts more effectively.

You can transform habitual patterns of responding to conflict. Start with you–*not* your boss and *not* your spouse. The person that angers you is not likely to change because you demand it, anyway. This chapter offers you exercises to develop your skills for working creatively with yourself and others with whom you experience conflict.

Effectiveness: Solving Interpersonal Problems

The rewards of understanding your responses to conflict and working with your vulnerabilities are powerful. Dr. David McClelland (1990), a psychologist at Boston University, is studying the impact of interpersonal attitudes on general health status. His work suggests that we have better health when we have strong interests in affiliation *simply for the sake of "being affiliated."* Additionally, health status is better for people who have confidence in their ability to respond to interpersonal stress occasioned by affiliation. People with a hostile and cynical outlook on the world are at risk for more physical illness and for premature death. However, human beings can learn to affiliate and trust others. These lessons will result in increased immune function and less illness (Kabat-Zinn, 1991).

Couples can learn new skills for solving problems. Improved problem-solving will result in greater marital satisfaction. Jacobson (1979, 1985) reports that distressed couples tend to make negative attributions about their partner's behavior. These negative interpretations pave the way for criticism of the partner rather than thoughtful evaluation of self. If we want high quality intimate relationships, we need to master psychological acceptance and behavioral change strategies in the difficult context of interpersonal relating. Use of a communication training book for couples may provide you with additional information and exercises to support your work in this critical area (Gottman, et al., 1976). At times, you may need to involve a counselor or psychologist to enhance your success in creating a high quality intimate relationship.

Goal Setting

Rate your present abilities in this area on the scales provided in the Goal Setting box. Use a relationship that is characterized by unresolved conflict as your reference for these ratings. Also, decide on a specific target to address in this relationship. For example, Leslie decided to target "discussing school work" (content target) with her teenager son (relationship target). Make your choices concerning content and relationship targets now. Then, make your ratings prior to starting the Skill Work section. As usual, circle numbers to indicate your confidence and ability levels and mark an "x" on the numbers corresponding to your goals.

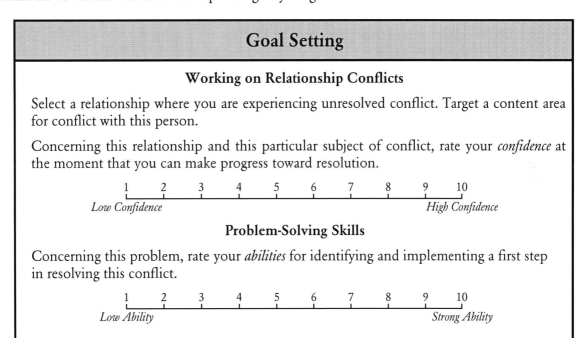

Goal Setting

Working on Relationship Conflicts

Select a relationship where you are experiencing unresolved conflict. Target a content area for conflict with this person.

Concerning this relationship and this particular subject of conflict, rate your *confidence* at the moment that you can make progress toward resolution.

```
    1    2    3    4    5    6    7    8    9    10
Low Confidence                              High Confidence
```

Problem-Solving Skills

Concerning this problem, rate your *abilities* for identifying and implementing a first step in resolving this conflict.

```
    1    2    3    4    5    6    7    8    9    10
Low Ability                                 Strong Ability
```

Skill Work: Responding to Interpersonal Conflict

Dancing provides a good metaphor for resolving interpersonal conflicts. There are at least three stages involved in learning to dance. The beginning phase involves knowing yourself well; the next phase involves connecting with another cooperatively, and the most advanced phase involves coordinated, complex movements. One cannot skip over phase one as it is imperative that you know yourself, accept yourself (both your strengths and weaknesses) and have confidence in your mental and physical readiness to dance. You need to feel a sense of kinship with your own breath, feelings, rhythms, and patterns. With this, you are ready to connect with a partner. Dancing begins in phase two and requires moving close to another and touching. How you and your partner connect is created by both of you and is fundamental to your next move, moment-to-moment, every day of your relationship. Dancing–whether the fox trot, the waltz, or the western swing–proceeds in directions that support the common goal of the dancers–to dance. Conflict need not stop the dance. Conflict can actually make the dance more interesting.

1. Beginning Exercises: Love, Respect and Trust

A. The Daily Care Moment Exercise

Stand with your hands facing in toward your abdomen. Extend your arms upward with your palms turned upward. Slowly, circle your arms out and down toward your sides. Allow your arms to continue in motion, flowing up again from the center of your body. Make large circles on both sides of your body. After making seven slow circles, reverse the direction of the circle and make seven more circles. Then, rest one hand on top of the other on your abdomen. As you do so, say to yourself, "I wrap myself in a warm blanket and allow myself to be." Allow yourself to generate feelings of kindness and love and direct them toward yourself. Spend several moments generating and breathing in care for yourself. When your mind wonders, you may redirect your awareness by suggesting, "I allow myself to be." If you like, you can continue with this exercise of generating loving feelings and extend the gift of these feelings to others.

B. Awareness of Personal Feelings

In order to communicate effectively, you need to be aware of your own feeling states. Spend a few minutes each day this week checking in with yourself emotionally. Ask yourself, "How do I feel right now?" This is actually more difficult than it may seem. Most of us are not accustomed to attending closely to feeling states. When you know and accept your own feeling states, you are in a stronger position to choose your response to conflict situations. You are less vulnerable to emotionally triggered reactions, which usually make conflict worse.

C. Respectful Expression of Feelings

When you know your own feelings, you can choose to experience them privately *or* to share them with another. Further, you can choose "how to" express your feelings. The best results come when you express your feelings in a way that is both respectful to yourself *and* the person with whom you have a conflict. Respectful expression is genuine and not intended to harm yourself or others. During the next week, watch closely when a conflict begins. Notice your feelings. Make a conscious decision about whether you will express your feelings. If you choose to make your feelings known to another, plan "how" to express them. Keep a record of these situations. If you are using the "Daily Wellness Check" approach, make your notes on conflicts throughout the day and your awareness and expression of feelings in your DW Check notebook. During quiet moments, re-evaluate your notes. Look at your options and practice making intentional choices concerning your expression of feelings. Allow yourself ample time to prepare for respectful expression.

2. Connecting Exercises: Joining and Defining the Direction of Dance

A. Caring Days Exercise

In 1980, Dr. Stuart suggested a Caring Days exercise to help couples in conflict increase their rate of daily positive interactions. This exercise is also useful in other relationship contexts, such as parent-child relationships. This procedure helps to create more positive feelings and provides a supportive environment for solving problems. Ask for your friend or loved one to cooperate. Both of you will need to write out a list of positive, specific, small behaviors you would like the other to do to *demonstrate her/his caring for you.* Your lists need to include behaviors that can be performed on a daily or weekly basis. Avoid requesting activities that have been the subject of recent conflicts. Next, exchange your lists. Offer a list of eight to ten behaviors, so that your partner can make choices. Ask any questions needed to clarify the behaviors requested of you. Each of you need to select at least five behaviors from the list. Share your choices. Once you come to an agreement on the caring behaviors, *commit* to performing the caring behaviors on an almost daily basis. You do not need to be *inspired* to engage in the behaviors–of course, that would be nice. You only need to do what you promised to do and to observe the value of this procedure for paving the way to effective problem-solving. Do *notice and express appreciation* when your friend or loved one engages in a caring behavior that you requested.

B. Aikido Blending Exercise

In *Full Catastrophe Living* (1991), Dr. Jon Kabat-Zinn suggests an Aikido exercise called "blending." This exercise may be of use to you in learning more about your patterns of responding to conflict. You may complete this exercise with a friend or loved one. As you implement the exercise, take time to feel all of the reactions in your mind and body. There are three exercises and two roles in each of the exercises. You will need to repeat each exercise twice so that each of you has an opportunity to experience each of the roles in the exercises. These exercises require you to be highly attentive to your body, thoughts, sensations, balance, and breath. Between the exercises, pause and discuss your results with each other. This will help deepen your experience and maximize your benefit from the exercise.

The three exercises are called the "door mat," the "attack-back," and "blending." All three involve the role of the attacker and the attacked. Be sure to repeat the exercises so that you have a chance to experience attacking and being attacked in all three movements. Refrain from talking during the movements. Focus your attention on your mind and body.

All three exercises start with you and your partner standing about four or five feet apart. The attacker role is always the same. The "attacker" extends both arms forward from the shoulders and walks towards the "attacked" partner, as if to connect with the "attacked" partner's shoulders and push them. The "attacker," of course, walks slowly and intends no real harm in the exercises.

In the "*door mat*" exercise, the "attacked" person responds to the "attacker" by lying down on the floor. Once you move into these positions, hold them for several minutes and explore your reactions.

In the "*attack-back*" exercise, the "attacked" person responds to the "attacker" by mirroring the "attacker's" movement. The "attacked" person raises her/his arms and moves toward the "attacker." The "attacker" and "attacked" engage with arms extended and pushing against each other's shoulders. Hold this position and study your responses.

In the "*blending*" exercise, the "attacked" person responds with the following sequence of behaviors.

- Steps one step forward and one step toward the side.

- Extends her/his hand to gently connect with one of the attacker's hands.

- Receives the energy of the attacker and *turns in the momentum* of his or her energy

- Now, faces the same direction as the attacker.

Once you are in this position, maintain it. As the "attacked" person, you avoided head-on impact, showed a willingness to connect and turned so that you could look at the perspective of the "attacker." Study your personal reactions in both roles. Notice the moment when you change from adversaries to partners in the blending exercise. Your ending position allows you and your partner many options for movement. The "attacker" is free to change agendas – or make a new step.

The "blending" exercise contrasts with the "door mat" and "attack-back" positions. Most people feel frustrated in both roles in the "door mat" position. The "attack-back" position is usually more satisfying. However, it becomes tiring or boring, as few other moves are viable from the ending stance. When you make the "blending" response, conflict becomes interesting.

3. Dancing Exercises: Steps in Solving Interpersonal Conflicts Skillfully

Jacobson and Margolin (1979) developed a problem-solving manual for couples. The manual outlines strategies for constructive conflict resolution. On-going practice of these skills, like ballroom or swing dancing on Friday nights, may be part of "having conflict well" in intimate relationships. The Jacobson and Margolin guidelines include the following:

a) *Set an Agenda.* Your agenda needs approval by both parties. Additionally, the agenda needs to be something that you can expect to complete in 30 to 60 minutes of problem solving.

b) *Positively and Specifically Define Problems.* Use "I" statements to help you maintain a position of responsibility for yourself. Avoid blaming. "I" statements are statements that express your beliefs, perceptions, wants, or feelings in an open, honest way. For example, you might make this "I" statement: "I am tired and cannot do my best problem-solving until I am more rested." "I" statements facilitate communication, while "you" statements often impede progress in problem-solving. The following are examples of "you" statements: "You always have to have your way;" or "You are trying to make me feel guilty." Once you define the problem, confirm that each of you agrees on all details of the definition.

c) *Discuss One Problem at a Time.* As a rule, address only one problem in each session of problem-solving. Gently remind each other when and if you start to get off track. Often a question, such as, "How is this related to the problem we are attempting to resolve?" is an adequate reminder to a partner who has lost focus.

d) *Focus on Solutions Instead of Blame.* Brainstorm solutions. Each person needs to generate possible solutions. Often, taking turns is a good procedure. Try to avoid screening solutions carefully. Some solutions can be "outrageous." Generate a list. After you have a list, evaluate each solution. Consider the advantages and disadvantages of each solution.

e) *Compromise.* Choose a solution that involves both parties winning something. The best solutions are win-win. Be clear about your choice. Write down the solution you select and set a specific time to evaluate the effectiveness of the solution.

Example: Solving Interpersonal Problems

David and Jill had been married for fifteen years. Their only child was 12. Both were working full-time and struggled with finding time to complete routine household tasks. Mail piled up and the dishes were sometimes left for days at a time. Jill did the laundry and resented being confronted with preparing evening meals in a dirty kitchen. She often served cereal and fruit to herself and her daughter and left David to fend for himself when the kitchen was dirty. Whenever the two attempted to plan a strategy for maintaining a more tidy household, both became defensive and moved quickly to an "I am right and you are wrong" agenda. Their daughter often ended their arguments by asking them to "just stop fighting." Both returned to their corners of their messy house feeling dissatisfied with their communication skills, their relationship, and their house.

David read this chapter and shared it with Jill. Both agreed to explore their individual ability to care for themselves through the "Daily Caring Exercise." After practicing this for a week, both wanted to try the "Caring Days" procedure for a week. As both were feeling more confident about their individual abilities and about the viability of the relationship, they then decided to enter into formal problem-solving concerning maintaining a more tidy household. Ultimately, the two selected the solution of hiring a housekeeper to come twice each month and to work together for three hours to prepare for the housekeeper's visit. Additionally, they decided to put their daughter in charge of kitchen clean-up on a daily basis.

Behavioral Health Plan: Responding to Interpersonal Conflict

This week's Behavioral Health Plan requires you to commit to practice one or more of the strategies for responding to interpersonal conflict. Most people will want to include practice of one of the "Beginning" Exercises, as these provide a necessary foundation for the "Connecting" and "Dancing" exercises. Indicate on your Behavioral Health Plan the exercise(s) you plan to practice and make a note concerning the details of where and when.

In the section on expressing values, choose an area of life where you are experiencing interpersonal conflict. Select a strategy for responding to interpersonal conflict that you understand and perceive as potentially helpful to you in this area of your life. For example, you might decide to use "Dancing" exercises to resolve a conflict with your spouse about finances. Alternatively, you might choose to use a "Beginning" exercise, such as the "Daily Caring Moment" in order to improve your "Images of a Better Future" if you are in a "glass ceiling" situation in your job and feel discouraged.

This Behavioral Health Plan may be particularly difficult to implement. Note your support person on the planning format. Plan a special reward for yourself. If your commitment is not high, consider changing your plan to involve one of the "Beginning" exercises. Give yourself a week to gain some momentum in this area and then advance to a more challenging exercise.

References

Beck, C. H., & Smith, S. (1993). *Nothing special: Living Zen*. New York, NY: Harper Collins Publishers.

DeShazer, S. (1991). *Putting difference to work*. New York, NY: W. W. Norton & Company.

Gottman, J., Notarius, C., Gonso, J., & Markman, H. (1976). *A couple's guide to communication*. Champaign, IL: Research Press.

Jacobson, J. S. (1984). A component analysis of behavioral marital therapy: The relative effectiveness of behavior exchange and problem-solving training. *Journal of Consulting and Clinical Psychology, 52*, 295-305.

Jacobson, N. S., & Gurman, A. S. (1986). *Clinical handbook of marital therapy*. New York: Guilford Press.

Jacobson, N. S., & Koerner, K. (1994). Emotional acceptance in integrative behavioral couple therapy. In S. C. Hayes, N. S. Jacobson, V. M. Follette, & M. J. Dougher (Eds.), *Acceptance and Change: Content and Context in Psychotherapy* (pp. 109-118). Reno, NV: Context Press.

Jacobson, N. S., & Margolin, G. (1979). *Marital therapy: Strategies based on social learning and behavior exchange principles*. New York: Brunner/Mazel.

Jacobson, N. S., McDonald, D. W., Follette, W. C., & Berley, R. A. (1985). Attributional processes in distressed and non-distressed married couples. *Cognitive Therapy and Research, 9*, 35-50.

Kabat-Zinn, J. (1991). *Full Catastrophe Living: Using the wisdom of your body and mind to face stress, pain, and illness*. New York, NY: Dell Publishing Group, Inc.

Montagu, A. (1986). *Touching: The human significance of the skin* (3rd Ed.). New York, NY: Harper.

Stuart, R. (1980). *Helping couples change: A social learning approach to marital therapy*. New York: Guilford Press.

Behavioral Health Plan

Strategies For Responding to Interpersonal Conflict

This week I will use the following exercises:

☐ BEGINNING EXERCISES   ☐ Daily Caring Moment

☐ Awareness of Personal Feelings

☐ Respectful Expression of Feelings

☐ CONNECTING EXERCISES   ☐ Caring Days

☐ Blending

☐ DANCING EXERCISES (actual formal practice of the guidelines)

Describe details concerning "where and when" you will apply the exercise(s) to solving an interpersonal conflict.

Strategies For Expressing Values

The area of life I will target for expressing my values is:

☐ Enjoying Things Alone   ☐ Sensual Experience

☐ Accomplishing Things Alone   ☐ Fun with Others

☐ Talking with Others   ☐ Images of a Better Future

☐ Contentment with Work

To increase my expression of my values in this area, I will:

When:	Where:

With whom:

Who will support my plan?

As a reward for following my Behavioral Health Plan, I will:

Am I 100% committed to this Plan?	☐ Yes ☐ No

Chapter 6

Expressing Yourself...
Assertively And Creatively

Weekly Review

Last week you started a program to increase your awareness of your patterns of responding to interpersonal conflict. I hope your work with these strategies will continue, as resolving conflicts with others is a critical aspect of learning to live life well. When you are more aware of yourself and your "hot buttons" in conflict situations, you can master techniques for resolving disputes more easily. Take a moment to assess your conflict resolution abilities on the scales in the Goal Attainment box.

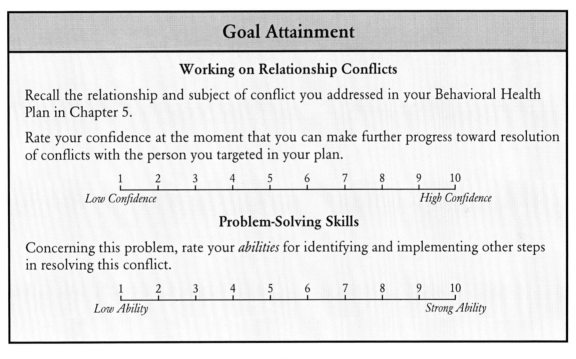

Did anyone in your life notice anything different about *you* as you went about implementing your Behavioral Health Plan last week? Loved ones will sometimes notice the influence of practicing the "Daily Caring Moment" exercise. The work of resolving conflict well is an on-going challenge for most people. Do continue to make a conscious, intentional effort. Depending on the results of your plan, you may want to continue to work with the same person and content area. Alternatively, you may be ready to change the content area or target person.

In this Chapter, you evaluate your abilities for expressing yourself assertively and creatively. You may have strong skills in one of these areas and weaker skills in the other. Strong skills in both areas prepare you for responding to difficulties in life with considerable psychological resilience. Evaluate your strengths and weaknesses. **Your may decide to focus on one area rather than both.**

Evaluate your overall progress using your standard self-assessment method and, then, assess your need for skill development in these two important areas.

Self-Assessment

Complete the method(s) of self-assessment that you chose to track your progress. You may photocopy the form(s) most useful to you from Appendix E. **If you are using the Quality of Life Scale** (QL Scale), check to see if your present ratings in the Emotional Experience and Behavioral Action areas differ from those obtained at the beginning of Chapter 5. The exercises suggested in Chapter 5 are quite powerful. Changes resulting from their application may be detected in the short-term, long-term or both. Since we are first and foremost social beings, successful application of skills for solving interpersonal conflict can have a tremendously positive impact on our sense of well-being.

For example, Jane decided to target "Contentment with Work." She and her supervisor had a history of conflict, and they tended to avoid each other. Both were generally effective in their roles. However, their unresolved conflict limited the creativity they could generate in collaborative endeavors and their individual enjoyment of being in the work environment. At the suggestion of her manager's supervisor, they agreed to use a mediator to improve their relationship. Jane began to practice the "Daily Caring Moment" exercise at the beginning of her work day. Additionally, she practiced the Aikido exercises with a close friend. During the "blending" exercise, she discovered that she found it difficult to *make the turn* and to view the attacker's perspective. This discovery helped her clarify the importance of attempting to *turn and see her supervisor's perspective*. Jane engaged in the daily caring moment just before the mediation meeting. She reminded herself to turn and see her supervisor's perspective during the meeting. While the tangible results of this initial meeting were few, Jane felt encouraged by her sense of calm during the session and her ability to understand more of her supervisor's viewpoint. She planned to continue to work to improve her relationship with her supervisor.

If you are using medications, the Symptoms Checklist may be useful to you in evaluating the completeness of your response to antidepressant medications (See Appendix E). By this point, you are probably noticing significant improvement in all of your initial symptoms. If you are still troubled by a particular symptom, discuss this with your physician.

If you are using the Daily Wellness Check (DW Check), what were your highest and lowest daily ratings during the past week? How did these two days differ? What key thoughts or activities occur on days when you "live life well?" Do you see themes that relate to interpersonal conflict and styles of problem solving? While Ralph did not like conflict, he noted that his ratings were higher on days when he did not avoid conflict. Like Jane, he identified the skill of "trying to see the other person's perspective" as an important aspect of solving conflicts. Take a moment to reflect on your DW ratings for the past week. Write down thoughts and activities in your life that are associated with a higher quality of life. Note observations that may help you plan additional behavioral change programs.

Discoveries from Daily Wellness Checks During the Past Week
1.
2.
3.
4.

If you have not used the Daily Wellness Check method in the past few weeks, consider using it for the next week. It is particularly useful as an adjunct to the strategies and skills covered in this chapter and can be incorporated into your life on an on-going basis once you "graduate" from this program.

Strategies: Personal Assertion and Creative Expression

In this chapter, I suggest cultivation of two strategies for expressing yourself and your values: personal assertion and creative expression. Personal assertion is a strategy that requires on-going practice of balance between respect and acceptance of *yourself **and*** respect and acceptance of *others*. Creative expression is the balancing of who you are with what you have to work with right now.

When you feel that your life is going well, you are most likely to be living in a state of balance. You approach your life creatively and your life reflects your values. You are making decisions. You are setting goals and working towards them. You are willing to have the problems you have and tend to see them as challenges rather than obstacles in your life. On a daily basis, your activities represent you putting your values into play. You are involved with others and with the world.

During difficult periods in life, we often become less balanced. Our fluctuation between "doing" and simply "being" looses balance. Western society encourages productivity. We may over-respond to this cultural message. At points in our lives, we may find ourselves waking in the morning with a startle and almost springing from our beds to *get busy*. Our days can be packed with *doing stuff* to show our importance to others, convince us momentarily of our goodness, distract us from the pain and anger of non-acceptance, and conceal our weakness from ourselves and others. Our lifestyles depart from what is truly important to us. Our quality of life suffers, and our health often declines.

The exercises presented in this chapter help you develop personal assertion skills and a pattern of regular participation in creative activities. We can respond to highly stressful life circumstances with assertion and without giving up outlets for creative expression. Throughout our lives, we can express our fundamental assertive rights and our creative potential.

Unfortunately, parts of our *training for adulthood* may lead us to needlessly concede expressive abilities of childhood. We can be forthright and valued by others. We can be productive and playful and creative–at the same time. When we know how to re-balance our lives, we can correct tendencies to please others at the expense of our own quality of life. We can change patterns of over-producing and over-achieving. Assertive and creative expression skills help us find balance in life so that our day-to-day "doing" does not take on a *driven* quality. When we forget to apply these important strategies for balancing our lives, we may respond to difficult life stresses by making a counter-intuitive move and driving ourselves to do *more*, produce *more*, and please *more rather than less*. Relaxation efforts may also become "driven."

Driven doing takes many forms–"channel surfing" on your television; redoubling your efforts to be a perfect mother, employee, child; turning up the radio when you start to feel empty and sad in your commute home from work; compulsive shopping, eating, reading; checking and rechecking your stove; blaming your parents, priest, or doctor. Your own particular garden of *driven doing* grows from your life experiences. Re-learning *balancing strategies,* including assertive and creative expression, prepares you to make value-based, conscious choices about what you do and what you leave undone.

You can learn to balance your life on a daily basis. When you are able to detect imbalances, you can apply psychological acceptance and behavioral change strategies. You can be yourself and do what "matters" to you in the world. Hayes and Strosahl (1996), experts on psychological acceptance, suggest that you feel vitally alive when you are committed to living what you value and willing to accept the feelings that come up in the process of doing what you value. Vitality and balance are closely related.

Balance requires skillfulness in validating yourself and others. Validation, whether of yourself or another, boosts autonomy (Linehan, 1993). Autonomy empowers you to act assertively and creatively. However critical you are of yourself or others, you can *make room* for this aspect of yourself, and *do what you value* in the world. You can think, "I am not good enough" and behave in ways that demonstrate a great deal of respect of self and others. You can think, "I'll never get this project done," and take time to play the flute (or crochet or golf or write a poem).

Daily practice of balancing skills is needed in order to sustain a high quality of life. Supportive counseling from a friend or professional may help develop skillfulness in these areas. King Solomon, a wise counselor to his people, understood how much his people suffered with balancing concerns about self with concerns about others and balancing productive work with creative activity. He understood the power of self-critical thoughts. After listening to a person's problem, King Solomon typically asked the person to read the inscription on his ring. The inscription read, *"This too shall pass."* You can learn to monitor yourself, accept painful thoughts, and find a day-to-day balance between working and playing, respecting yourself and respecting others.

In order to live assertively and creatively, we need to re-evaluate our lives and our resources on a continual basis. The nature of effective assertion and satisfying creative expression often changes during the course of a lifetime. "Simply being while doing" may take many forms–a child making mud pies, a person washing dishes, a human being walking with a pet dog.

Ram Doss tells a story of a talk he gave on meditation in Seattle, Washington in the late 1960's. He explains that most of the people who came to his talks at that time had long hair, wore jeans or flowing garments, smelled of patchouli, and were under 30 years of age. At this particular talk, an older woman, 60-something, stood out for him when he scanned the audience prior to starting his talk. His eyes returned often to study this curious participant who was clad in a stripped polyester dress and wearing a large straw hat with a flower on top. After the talk, he sought out the woman. She smiled at him and said, "Oh, thank you very much." He responded, "You are welcome, but did you understand what I was saying in my talk about balance, meditation and states of consciousness? Did my talk make sense to you?" She clasped her hands together in front of her chest and explained, "Oh, yes, Mr. Ram Doss," I understand perfectly, "You see–I knit." Artistic activities are rich with possibilities for cultivation of mental states characterized by *"simply being while doing."*

Effectiveness: Personal Assertion and Creative Expression

Personal assertion skills form the basis of your ability to make direct, honest statements and to stand up for your rights (Lazarus, 1979). Effective assertion improves satisfaction with interpersonal relationships in all areas of life. Assertion skills empower adults to develop and maintain an intimate relationship (Beck, 1988). Additionally, parenting is more rewarding when adults have strong assertion skills (Gordon, 1970). In general, lower levels of assertion are associated with higher levels of neuroticism and more problems with mental functioning (Gilbert & Allan, 1994). Furthermore, development of effective assertion skills may improve mood, hopefulness, and energy for enjoying life (Sanchez, et al., 1980).

Assertiveness training may be particularly important for women. Females may receive less support for assertion than males during childhood (Jakubowski-Spector, 1973). Lack of effective assertion skills may limit one's success in work environments as well as in personal relationships (Phelps & Austin, 1975). When we do not know how to assert our wants to others, we are left waiting for them to notice or to guess what our desires are. This is risky because others tend to be busy "doing" and are often caught in the language games of their own minds. Being more passive in our style of expression leaves us in a position of dependency. If we take a position of passivity habitually and without perceiving a choice to behave otherwise, we are susceptible to a myriad of psychological and physical problems.

Creative expression is closely related to effective personal assertion. Direct, open, honest, and forthright expression of thoughts and feelings provides a fertile environment for creativity. Most people are more satisfied with work environments that support assertive communication, autonomous decision-making, and creative expression. Autonomy is the perfect fertilizer for creativity, and creative expression *feels good*. In Dr. Maslow's personality theory, creative expression is a human need in the upper levels of the human development hierarchy. There is a richness available in creative experience that may be lacking in more basic levels of developmental experience, and this richness probably contributes significantly to productivity in work environments, as well as overall quality of life.

Creative expression supports development of a mental state that is restful and restorative. Lack of creative expression activities may contribute to problems in immune system functioning. Up to 16% of the variation we have in our natural killer cytotoxicity values is related to a sense of "un-wellness" associated with discouragement. Related symptoms include lowered energy and sleep disturbance (Cover & Irwin, 1994). Daily creative experiencing is good for your mental and physical health.

Goal Setting

Reflect for a moment on your present abilities in personal assertion and creative expression. Use the scales in the Goal Setting box to assess your abilities. Your assertion skills may depend on the interpersonal context. For example, you may be more assertive with your spouse than your supervisor. Your rating needs to represent an *average for all areas of your life at present*. Concerning creative expression, rate your frequency of expression. Everyone is capable of creative expression. We vary in the extent to which creative expression is integrated into our daily lives. Circle the number to indicate your ability or frequency. Mark an "x" on the numbers you select as your goals.

Goal Setting

Personal Assertion

Rate your ability to *assertively express* yourself in all areas of your life *on average* at the present moment.

```
    1    2    3    4    5    6    7    8    9    10
Low Ability                                  Strong Ability
```

Creative Expression

Use this rating scale to indicate how often you engage in creative activities.

```
    1    2    3    4    5    6    7    8    9    10
  Rarely                                       Daily
```

Skill Work: Assertive and Creative Expression

The skills involved in assertive and creative expression overlap. This section offers you exercises to help you assess your skills in both areas. Considering your results, you may decide to focus *on one or both* of these skill areas in your Behavioral Health Plan for the week.

Skill Work: Assertive Expression

Jakubowski and Lange (1978) provide the following definition of assertive behavior.

> "standing up for your assertive rights and expressing what you believe, feel, and want in direct, honest, appropriate ways that respect the rights of the other person (p. 2)."

This definition suggests that there are two basic components to effective assertion. These are: (1) knowing and believing your assertive rights, and (2) engaging in behaviors that are consistent with your rights. Bloom, Coburn and Pearlman (1975) suggested a long list of "Basic Assertive Rights." Ten basic assertive rights are listed in the Assertive Assessment exercise. This exercise will help you assess your present level of development in the area of assertive expression.

Exercise: Assertive Expression Self-Assessment

Review the ten basic assertive rights listed in the Assertive Assessment Exercise box on page 79. In column I, rate the strength of your belief concerning each of the rights. Use a rating scale where 1 = a weak belief and 10 = a strong belief. In column II, rate the extent to which your day-to-day life reflects a strong belief in each of the rights. If you have a weak belief regarding a particular right, your rating concerning acting on the belief will probably be low. We tend to behave according to our beliefs. Therefore, your initial efforts to improve assertive expression skills need to address weak beliefs. Brief half-day assertiveness training workshops may be helpful to you in further clarifying and strengthening your belief in specific assertive rights. Most people benefit from talking with others who have somewhat stronger beliefs in a particular area. As your beliefs become stronger, you are more ready to make plans to increase your ratings in column II. The following exercise (Assertive Plan) will help you express your beliefs in day-to-day life.

Exercise: Assertive Plan

Even when your beliefs in a specific assertive right are strong, behavioral expression can be very difficult. Joining an Assertive Training group or class provides a place to practice behavioral expression, as well as re-evaluate basic rights that you give yourself and others. If you have a strong belief in one or more of the ten assertive rights and your life does not reflect this belief, use the following steps to help you align your behavior with your belief. After reviewing these steps, use the Assertive Plan Worksheet on page 80 to develop a plan.

Step One: Identify A Target Situation.

Identify several situations where the right applies and your behavior does not reflect your belief in this right. Organize these situations in a list. Arrange them according the difficulty you would have in changing your behavior. Start your list with the easiest situation. The situation where you could change your behavior most easily will be your initial target for change. You can return to item two on your list later.

Step Two: Define the Desired Outcome.

Define what you want to see happen in this situation. Formulate this as your desired outcome.

Step Three: Set a Behavioral Goal.

Clarify what you want your own behavior in this situation to look like. Write out specific statements that you would like to make in the situation.

Step Four: Imagine and Plan for "Zings."

Take time to imagine the situation in detail. "See" yourself engaging in the desired assertive behavior. Also, imagine the "zings" or problematic interactions that could distract you from behaving assertively. Imagine that you accept the zings and continue to demonstrate your goal behavior. Imagine also that the desired outcome does develop.

Assertive Assessment Exercise		
I. Strength of Your Belief*	**II. Lived In Day-To-Day Life****	**III. Basic Assertive Rights**
		1. The right to act in ways that promote your dignity and self-respect as long as others' rights are not violated in the process.
		2. The right to say no and not feel guilty.
		3. The right to be treated with respect.
		4. The right to experience and express your feelings.
		5. The right to take time to slow down and think.
		6. The right to change your mind.
		7. The right to ask for what you want.
		8. The right to do less than you are humanly capable of doing.
		9. The right to ask for information.
		10. The right to make mistakes.
		11. The right to feel good about yourself.

*Use a rating scale, where 1 = a weak belief and 10 = a strong belief.
** Use a rating scale, where 1 = not lived in day-to-day life and 10 = lived in day-to-day life.

Assertive Plan Worksheet

Step One: Identify a Target Situation.

Step Two: Define the Desired Outcome.

Step Three: Set Behavioral Goals.

1.

2.

Step Four: Imagine and Plan for Zings.

Possible Zing	Plan

Step Five: Make a Practice Plan.

I will practice with   on

Step Six: Do It and Specify a Reward for Yourself.

When:	Where:

With Whom:

Reward:

Step Seven: Evaluate and Describe the Results. Pretend that you are a scientist. Look at your results objectively. Continue working toward the solution or goal by simply determining and planning a next step or by going through these seven steps again.

Anticipated Result	Actual Result	Discrepancy

Next step(s):

Step Five: Practice.

Actively practice the behavior you want to perform in this situation. Recruit a friend to practice with you if possible. If this is not feasible, use your pet or your mirror as a "witness" of your efforts to develop assertive expression skills.

Step Six: Do it.

You know this step from your problem-solving skills review. Remember, you do not need to feel confident or relaxed or inspired to "do it." Fortunately, you only have to "do it."

Step Seven: Evaluate your Results.

Carefully review what happened. Acknowledge what you liked about your behavior and the results of the interaction. Also, think about changes you might make in the future.

After evaluating your results you can return to Step 1 and address the second item on your list. You will develop facility as you use this 7-step procedure repeatedly. Use the Assertive Plan Worksheet to develop a plan. Remember to start with a somewhat easy situation.

Example: Assertive Expression

Pamela was a mid-level manager in a grocery warehouse. She had worked in numerous positions with the company over the past 14 years. She had always been a hard worker. The company valued her reliability and high standards. They asked a lot of her when a strike occurred, and the strike left Pam with numerous symptoms of "burn out." She re-evaluated her priorities in life and took a closer look at her job and the stress at work. When she evaluated her response to the list of Basic Assertive Rights, she recognized several discrepancies between her beliefs and her actions at work. First, she realized that she did believe she had "the right to do less than she was humanly capable of doing" at work. However her behavior at work rarely reflected this belief. Second, she noticed that she did give herself the right to make mistakes. She wanted to strengthen this belief and practice it in her behavior.

Pamela decided to start a behavioral health plan to improve her assertive expression skills and to focus on her work setting. Pamela specified Friday morning meetings as her target situation for assertive expression. In Friday morning meetings, mid-level managers reported productivity statistics and received special project assignments. Pamela identified several desired outcomes for the next meeting. These included the following.

> The supervisor will acknowledge my decision to volunteer for only one project assignment each week (as this is the expectation for all managers).

> The supervisor will accept that I will be a few hours late in completing calculations for the productivity ratio.

The plan was challenging for Pamela. She practiced her planned assertive responses with a close friend, who supported her belief and behavioral change program. Pamela visualized her success in preparation for the meeting. Additionally, she wrote out a behavioral goal. Her goal was to make the following two assertive statements during the meeting.

> I want to see more equitable assignment of special projects in this group.
>
> I do not have the productivity ratio statistic prepared. I will e-mail it to you later today.

Writing these goals on paper prior to the meeting helped Pamela to feel calm and ready to demonstrate these new behaviors. The person conducting the meeting asked her to take a second project assignment, and she declined. In a calm, clear voice, Pam stated her initial request, "I want to see more equitable assignment of special projects in this group." While appearing surprised, the meeting leader accepted Pamela's refusal without an argument and actually supported her request for more equality in project assignments. Further, the leader only nodded when Pam indicated that she had not completed one of the statistics for her report. Pamela felt somewhat nervous. She worked with her breathing to relax herself. At the end of the meeting, she experienced a great deal of personal satisfaction in having expressed herself in a way that was consistent with her beliefs.

Skill Work: Creative Expression

Creative expression is more of an attitude than an activity. When you express yourself creatively, you lose yourself to your work and enter the serenity of the moment. Some people experience creative expression in gardening; others prefer singing or dancing. Still others may find more satisfaction in drawing, painting, or working with clay. In creative expression, the attitude is one of focused play using readily-available opportunities. Although a *product* may be planned, the *process* of creative expression is non-competitive and non-task focused. Our creative work "just looks (or feels or sounds or smells) the way it does" and "takes as much of our time as it does."

Exercise: Creative Expression Assessment

Most of us have activities that provide outlets for creative expression. However, we may give these activities up in order to address the needs of others or obtain a higher level of achievement in our careers. In the Creative Expression Assessment exercise, evaluate the overall presence of creative expression activities in your life at present. In column I, list your favorite creative expression activities. In column II, indicate the number of hours you spent engaging in each of these activities during the *past week*.

Creative Expression Assessment	
I. Creative Expression Activity	**II. # of Hours Engaged in Activity in Past Week**

Exercise: Create Expression Plan

If you had difficulty identifying five creative expression activities, take time to evaluate your gifts or interests. Also, consider the resources or potential materials in your life at the present moment. You may have many gifts: a strong sense of observation, good visual-motor coordination, flexibility, a nice voice, musical talent, good gross motor coordination, a keen sense

of color. Which of your talents agree with your current interests? Do you have additional assets? Our resources for creativity change over time. During high school, a person may access a gym for practicing dance movements. During child-rearing years, the same person, may discover the creative potential of jogging behind a stroller while singing baby songs. In older years, this person may take a bus to a trail head for a long nature walk. What resources are you using? What other resources are available to you? How can you incorporate creative activities into your daily routine? In your Behavioral Health Plan, you will have an opportunity to plan an initial experiment in this important area.

Example: Creative Expression

Fred was disabled by a work accident. He left his job as a construction worker at age 50, after 30 year of continual and satisfying employment. In his free time, Fred had always enjoyed carpentry projects in his home workshop. His hobbies included making furniture and upholstery. His disability was due to a back injury. His injury now blocked his pursuit of both work and leisure activities. Fred's life was void of activities for creative expression, and his opportunities for socializing were limited. Fred evaluated his "gifts." His visual-motor coordination was good; his sense of spatial design was strong; his vision was good. Many of his friends and relatives noted the artistic beauty and attention to detail in furniture he made before his injury. His limitations were his physical strength and flexibility. Fred looked at his resources. He discovered two possibilities: a lot of wood scraps and a sister who was a carver. Fred called his sister and discussed carving. The sister invited Fred to visit her for a week of instruction in carving and Fred agreed. He found that he enjoyed carving and that the physical demands of carving were within his physical abilities *and* utilized many of his strengths and resources. Fred decided to take a course in carving at an art school near his home so that he could continue to learn. He purchased a notebook and started drawing small animals that he would eventually learn to carve.

Behavioral Health Plan: Assertive and Creative Expression

This chapter includes two formats for your Behavioral Health Plan. Use the format that provides a structure for the strategy you plan to strengthen – Assertive *or* Creative Expression. If you plan to address Assertive Expression, complete the Assertive Expression Assessment and make an Assertive Expression Plan. Indicate who supports your becoming more assertive on the planning format. Talk with your support person several times this week concerning your assessment, plan, and results. If you select Creative Expression as your target, use the Behavioral Health Plan for Creative Expression Strategies. Indicate when you will complete the Creative Expression Assessment. Summarize your plan. Try to make the plan simple. Examples of creative expression plans include the following:

- "Visit the tropical fish store on Thursday and stay as long as I like"
- "Make a place on my desk for drawing materials on Monday and draw 20 minutes at lunch on Tuesday."
- "Sing in the shower every morning this week."
- "Find my last cross-stitch project and start stitching this Saturday – and listen to Mozart while I stitch."

In the Strategies for Expressing Values section, choose an area of your life that you have not yet addressed in the program. You have reviewed many strategies and you are probably ready to plan to express more of what is important to you in all areas of your life.

References

Beck, A. T. (1988). *Love is never enough*. New York: Harper & Row.

Bloom, L. Z., Coburn, K., & Pearlman, J. (1975). *The new assertive woman*. New York: Delacorte Press.

Cover, H., & Irwin, M. (1994). Immunity and depression: Insomnia, retardation, and reduction of natural killer cell activity. *Journal of Behavioral Medicine, 17*(2), 217-223.

de Shazer, S. (1991). *Putting Difference to Work*. New York, NY: W.W. Norton & Company.

Gilbert, P., & Allan, S. (1994*)*. Assertiveness, submissive behaviour and social comparison. *Journal of Clinical Psychology, 33*(3), 295-306.

Gordon, J. (1970). *Parent effectiveness training*. New York: Wyden Books.

Hayes, S. C., Strosahl, K. D., & Wilson, K. G. (1995). *Acceptance and commitment therapy: An experiential approach to behavior change*. New York, NY: Guilford Press.

Hayes, S. C. (1987). A contextual approach to therapeutic change. In N. S. Jacobson (Ed.), *Psychotherapists in clinical practice* (pp. 326-378). New York, NY: Guilford Press.

Jakubowski, P., & Lange, A. J. (1978). *The assertive option: Your rights and responsibilities*. Champaign, IL: Research Press Company.

Jakubowski-Spector, P. (1973). Facilitating the growth of women through assertive training. *The Counseling Psychologist, 4*, 75-86.

Lazarus, A. A. (1973). On assertive behavior: A brief note. *Behavior Therapy, 4*, 697-699.

Lewinsohn, P. M., Munoz, R. F., Youngren, M. A., & Zeiss, A. M. (1986). *Control your depression, Revised and updated*. New York, NY: Prentice Hall.

Linehan, M. M. (1993). *Skills training manual for treating borderline personality disorder*. New York, NY: Guilford Press.

Maslow, A. H. (1968). *Toward a psychology of being* (2nd Ed.). New York: Van Nostrand Reinhold.

Phelps, S., & Austin, N. (1975). *The assertive woman*. San Luis Obispo, CA: Impact Press.

Sanchez, V. C., Lewinsohn, P. M., & Lorson, D. (1980). Assertion training: Effectiveness in the treatment of depression. *Journal of Clinical Psychology, 36*, 526-529.

Zeiss, A. M., Lewinsohn, P. M., & Munoz, R. F. (1979). Nonspecific improvement effects in depression using interpersonal, cognitive and pleasant effects focused treatments. *Journal of Consulting and Clinical Psychology, 47*, 427-439.

Behavioral Health Plan
Strategies For Assertive Expression
I will complete the Assertiveness Assessment Exercise on: (date).
I will complete an Assertiveness Plan Worksheet on: (date).
The person who supports me in becoming assertive is:
I will ask her or him to give me an opportunity to practice assertive responses prior to implementing my plan.   ☐ Yes   ☐ No
I will implement my Assertiveness Plan on   (date) and evaluate it on   (date).
Strategies For Expressing Values
The area of life I will target for expressing my values is: ☐ Enjoying Things Alone   ☐ Sensual Experience ☐ Accomplishing Things Alone   ☐ Fun with Others ☐ Talking with Others   ☐ Images of a Better Future ☐ Contentment with Work
To enhance my expression of values in this area, I will:

When:	Where:

With whom:
Who will support my plan?
As a reward for following my Behavioral Health Plan, I will:
Am I 100% committed to this Plan?   ☐ Yes   ☐ No

Behavioral Health Plan
Strategies For Creative Expression
I will complete the Creativity Assessment on: (date).
My Creativity Plan is:
I will implement my Creativity Plan from   to   and evaluate it on   (date).
Strategies For Expressing Values

The area of life I will target for expressing my values is:

☐ Enjoying Things Alone   ☐ Sensual Experience

☐ Accomplishing Things Alone   ☐ Fun with Others

☐ Talking with Others   ☐ Images of a Better Future

☐ Contentment with Work

To enhance my expression of values in this area, I will:

When:	Where:
With whom:	
Who will support my plan?	
As a reward for following my Behavioral Health Plan, I will:	
Am I 100% committed to this Plan? ☐ Yes ☐ No	

Chapter 7

Continuing To Live Life Well:
Planning Your Lifestyle

If you are pursing the "Basic Program," you have just completed a Behavioral Health Plan to help you solve a difficult life problem. Respond to the scaling questions in the Goal Attainment box at the start of Chapter 5 to evaluate your progress. Consider your results and plan further. You can solve huge problems one step at a time.

If you are completing the "Enhanced Program," your last Behavioral Health Plan helped you further develop your skills in assertive or creative expression (or both). Evaluate your progress and continue your efforts to solve interpersonal conflicts well and to express yourself effectively and creatively. These skills will buffer the impact of negative stress.

In reading this book, you have experimented with a wide array of coping strategies. You are probably recognizing daily benefits from using these strategies. In this last chapter, I invite you to reflect on your experiences thus far and to plan a lifestyle that supports your discoveries about your values and coping. Your lifestyle is the totality of your day-to-day pattern of living on a year-to-year basis. Your lifestyle is the "form" for your life and it needs to support your "purpose" in life. In this chapter, you will learn how to plan your lifestyle and to continue your use of key strategies. Research suggests that *continued planning* is critical in order to strengthen new changes in behavior.

Self-Assessment

Complete the method(s) of self-assessment that you choose to track your progress. Compare your results and note your progress. Hopefully, self-assessment is becoming a part of your life on a weekly or even daily basis.

Which assessment methods have worked best for you during the past 6 to 8 weeks? Which method was easier for you to complete? Which approach gave you the information you needed for planning and evaluating of your progress? Take a moment to write down your knowledge concerning assessment strategies and their applicability in your life right now. Use the Discoveries box to summarize your experience and plan for the future. Commit to a method of self-assessment for monitoring your progress during the next *six months*.

Strategies: Planning for the Future

Coping skills, rather than stress, itself, define the quality of a person's life. Suzanne Kobasa and her colleagues (Kobasa, et al., 1985, 1983, 1982; Kobasa & Hilker, 1982) studied many different kinds of people, who lead highly stressful lives. She found that certain psychological characteristics protect people from stress. Dr. Kobasa refers to people who are rarely ill as "psychologically hardy." "Psychologically hardy" individuals consistently demonstrate the following three characteristics. The **Quality of Life Scale** assesses these characteristics in different terms.

Discoveries from Experience with Self-Assessment Method(s)	
My favorite assessment approach is: (Mark One or More)	☐ The Quality of Life Scale ☐ The Symptoms Checklist ☐ The Daily Wellness Check
My discoveries concerning self-assessment include: 	
I plan to continue with this approach to assessment during the next 6 months. (Mark One or More)	☐ The Quality of Life Scale ☐ The Symptoms Checklist ☐ The Daily Wellness Check

1. **Challenge (*Emotional Experience* on the QL Scale)**

   Hardy individuals see stress as challenging rather than overwhelming. They are ready and willing to experience their response to stress. They accept feelings of fear and sadness. The psychological orientation of "accepting the challenge" corresponds to the "*Emotional Experience*" area of The Quality of Life Scale.

2. **Control (Using *Coping Strategies* on the QL Scale)**

   Hardy individuals believe that they can influence their own surroundings. They are high in self-efficacy. Whatever the challenge, they believe that they can cope with it. The "control" orientation corresponds to the "*Using Coping Strategies*" area of The Quality of Life Scale.

3. **Commitment (*Living Your Values* on the QL Scale)**

   Hardy individuals feel fully involved in what they are doing on a daily basis. They give their activities their best effort. This "best effort" quality is associated with the "*Living Your Values*" section of The Quality of Life Scale.

The weekly Behavioral Health Plan is an effective format for maintaining and further improving your psychological hardiness. I encourage you to continue to use this format on a regular basis for the next six months. I also encourage you to continue to use other acceptance and change strategies suggested in this book. A common mistake is to think we only have to pay attention when things are *not going well*. In reality, you enable your life to continue to reflect your values by staying aware and making intentional choices *moment to moment*. Skillfully applying your coping strategies fuels self-efficacy and your energy for persevering.

Without a doubt, you will take a few steps backwards in the next few months. It is *very easy* to fall back into anger, rage, blaming and vindictiveness (Ellis, 1990). The strategy of accepting yourself, others, and painful conditions that you cannot change is difficult to *achieve momentarily*, never mind maintain on a long-term basis. You will dislike yourself at times. You will dislike others at times. This is qualitatively different from chronically raging against yourself or warring with others. The key to continued progress is awareness. Awareness occurs more often when you assess your progress on a regular basis.

More strategic assessment is necessary when life presents "big" challenges. Dr. Peter Lewinsohn, a psychologist at the University of Oregon, suggests that the following stressful events require more focused self-assessment and planning efforts to avoid "slippage" from a desired lifestyle.

1. **Social Separations**

   These include death of a loved one, as well as divorce. Additionally, a child leaving home constitutes a social separation. Finally, moving to a new home entails multiple separation experiences.

2. **Health-Related Events**

   Personal injury and diagnosis of a medical illness constitute health-related events. A flare-up in management of a chronic disease may also occasion "slippage" from a planned style of living. Certainly, the illness or injury of a loved one impacts lifestyle. People caring for a loved one with Alzheimer's are highly vulnerable to negative lifestyle change and onset of symptoms of depression.

3. **New Roles**

   Assuming a new role requires multiple behavior changes. Examples of new roles include marriage or birth of a child. While these roles may be desirable, they require major changes to daily life.

4. **Work-Related Events**

   These events include obtaining a new job, a promotion or having significant changes made to your job description. Ending training or educational preparation for employment is another example of a work-related event that challenges one's lifestyle. Of course, retirement involves a major transition and requires careful planning concerning day-to-day living.

5. **Financial and Property Events**

   Financial problems may require one to make substantial changes. Destruction or theft of one's property is often sudden, yet can result in significant on-going negative change to one's lifestyle. Legal problems, of course, also impact one's commitment to a value-based style of living.

Living a lifestyle that reflects your values requires anticipation of stressful events and strategic planning. Some events can be anticipated. Other troubles in life arrive without warning. When you find yourself discouraged, remember that personal development is much like the evolution of a caterpillar into a butterfly. With human beings, the metamorphosis in on-going. Beck (1994) suggests that humans repeat the cycle of entering into the cocoon many times during a lifetime. Darker moments of life have meaning and value when we reflect, assess, and plan. When you find yourself distressed and discouraged, take time to "pull in" and "be still." Your evolution to a period of greater beauty and freedom is through the *respectful experience* of your anger, fear and sadness *and strategic planning* during cocoon phases of your development.

Effectiveness: Continuing to Live Life Well

You are most likely to continue to use strategies from this book if they become a part of your lifestyle. In research on the approaches recommended in this book, we found that people who remained "intentional" in their use of selected strategies for six months benefited more than people who made no concerted effort to follow a behavioral plan after "graduating" from these educational materials.

One of the most critical strategies to continue during the next six months is self-assessment. Continuing to live life well requires that you *attend* to your mind, body, and behavior on a regular basis. With on-going assessment, you are prepared to cope actively and immediately with stress. Active, strategic coping empowers you to *make gains* in personal development even during the most adverse circumstances. Strategic coping relies on your being aware of your behavior, so that you catch the first "wrong turn."

The reward of planing a lifestyle that promotes psychological hardiness is greater health and more resistance to illness and disease. Regular exercise and a strong social support group are associated with good health (Kobasa et al., 1982). A psychologically hardy lifestyle involves many opportunities for "connecting" with others. Our affiliation may be with pets or plants, as well as people. Trust in others and affiliative behaviors are qualities that "grow good corn" on the field of life (McClelland et al., 1985; McClelland, 1989; McClelland et al., 1991).

Goal Setting

Skill Work in this Chapter will help you start the process of planning your lifestyle. Use the scaling questions in the Goal Setting box to assess your commitment to incorporating helpful strategies from this book into your lifestyle. On-going implementation of your plan requires a strong commitment. If you find that your commitment is not strong and you have not progressed as much as you would like in reading this book, consider a different goal. Consider formulating a goal of seeking consultation with a psychologist or counselor. An expert may be able to help you very quickly. Invest the time and effort to do what is necessary to create a good life for yourself. Make your ratings now and place a note on your calendar to make another rating on these scaling items six months from today. Your goal is to behave according to the intention and commitment levels you mark below, assuming that they are above 6.

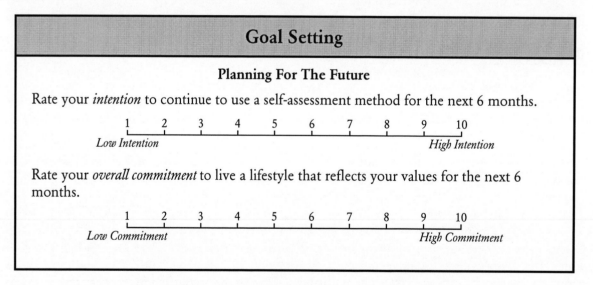

Skill Work: Continuing to Live Life Well

This chapter concludes by asking you to formulate a "Progress Plan" rather than a Behavioral Health Plan. The Progress Plan is a behavioral plan that summarizes your efforts to create and live the lifestyle you want during the next six months. The following two exercises will help you prepare to develop your Progress Plan. Complete the following exercises thoughtfully. Your work will provide a record for you to consult during difficult moments in the future.

Review of Strategies Exercise				
Instructions: Take time to complete this exercise carefully. Column 2 describes 20 strategies introduced in this book. In column 3, indicate the extent to which each of the strategies are *helpful to you* at this time. Use a rating scale where 1 = not helpful and 10 = very helpful. In column 4, indicate your intention to continue to use each of the strategies by marking an "X" in the *yes* or *no* box.				

1. Chapter	2. Strategy	3. Helpfulness to You (From 1 to 10)	4. Plan to Use	
			Y	N
I. Hoping...Planning... Doing	Generating hope by revising your explanation of your situation......................	_____	☐	☐
	Making a written Behavioral Health Plan ...	_____	☐	☐
II. Attending Your Mind And Making Value-Based Choices	Identifying psychological experiences you avoid..	_____	☐	☐
	Choosing a method of self-observation	_____	☐	☐
	Practicing the BOSE exercise	_____	☐	☐
	Using acceptance procedures in daily life ...	_____	☐	☐
III. Appreciating Your Mind And Body	Awareness/Concentration exercises.............	_____	☐	☐
	Imagery techniques......................................	_____	☐	☐
	Cultivating psychological neoteny	_____	☐	☐
IV. Solving Problems	Applying steps of formal problem-solving to a difficult situation in life	_____	☐	☐
V. Responding To Interpersonal Conflicts	Daily Caring Moment Exercise	_____	☐	☐
	Awareness of feelings..................................	_____	☐	☐
	Respectful expression of feelings	_____	☐	☐
	Caring Days	_____	☐	☐
	Blending exercise..	_____	☐	☐
	Use of formal guidelines for conflict resolution..	_____	☐	☐
VI. Expressing Yourself	Strengthening beliefs in basic assertive rights	_____	☐	☐
	Strengthening practice of basic assertive rights	_____	☐	☐
	Identifying creative expression activities	_____	☐	☐
	Practicing creative expression activities	_____		

Exercise: A Review of strategies

You have covered a lot of information and practiced many skills in the past few weeks. Completing the Review of Strategies Exercise will help you summarize your experience and plan for the future. Take time to complete this exercise carefully. Your work will provide a record for you to consult during difficult moments in the future. Column 1 provides the Chapter number and name, so that you can locate any strategies that you want to review easily. Column 2 describes 20 strategies introduced in this book. In column 3, indicate the extent to which each of the strategies was *helpful to you*. Use a rating scale where 1 = not helpful and 10 = very helpful. In column 4, indicate your intention to continue to use each of the strategies.

Exercise: Values

During the past few weeks, you have developed and implemented numerous Behavioral Health Plans with the goal of expressing your values in all key areas of your life. You will perhaps find the following exercise to be easier to complete than it was when you first tried it in the Introduction to the book. Complete the Values Exercise now. Your answers will help you in creating a lifestyle that reflects your values. Another approach to identifying values is to answer this question: *"If I were to die tomorrow, what would I want others to remember about my life?"*

Values Exercise
My most important values in life are:

Exercise: A Lifestyle that Mirrors my Values

Do your daily activities reflect what you value most? Perhaps you will say "yes" for some areas and "no" for others. The Lifestyle and Values Exercise will help you identify areas that will benefit from your attention and planning during the next six months. In the first column, list the values you recorded in the Values Exercise. In the second column, list one or more your activities that reflect each of your values. Mark columns 3 and 4 to indicate how often you have actually engaged in these activities over the past month. Which values have not been supported by your activities, at least weekly, during the past month? Plan to engage in more of these low-rate activities to *shape up* your lifestyle.

Lifestyle and Values Exercise			
Value	Activity	Daily	Weekly

Exercise: A Plan to Live a Value-Based Life

A final exercise will help you consolidate your discoveries from your previous Behavioral Health Plans. Please take the time to complete this exercise. It will help you develop a solid Progress Plan *and* be available to you should you begin to slip and need a quick reminder concerning your *planned* lifestyle.

Look back momentarily at your previous Behavioral Health Plans. Look specifically at the areas of your life that you have targeted. The Behavioral Health Plan to Live a Value-Based Life provides a format for you to use in recording your discoveries. Column 1 lists the seven areas of life that you may have targeted in behavioral health plans while using this workbook. Review these and, in column 2, record specific plans for each area for the next six months. Write in activities that you have found to increase your quality of life in each area. If you have not addressed all seven areas in previous plans, make an initial plan for areas of your life you have not yet addressed.

A Behavioral Health Plan to Live a Value-Based Life	
In living life well, I will:	My Plan
1. Enjoy moments alone by doing things like	
2. Set and accomplish goals	
3. Talk with others in ways that are consistent with my values	
4. Create moments of contentment in my work	
5. Experience life with my mind *and* body, enjoying all of my senses, by engaging in activities I value	
6. Be present and take time to have fun and be playful with others by doing things like	
7. Cultivate an attitude of acceptance toward negative feelings and images and know that painful moments, like enchanting experiences, will come and go.	
I plan to review this commitment:	☐ daily ☐ weekly ☐ monthly
I am 100% committed to this Plan	☐ Yes ☐ No
I will share my plan with:	

Exercise: Who is Your Buddy?

You are more likely to stay with a healthy, personally-meaningful lifestyle if you have support from others. In fact, a high quality of living requires reliable sources of social support. Do your present friends support your lifestyle? Will they support changes that you plan to make? If not, make adjustments in your network of friends.

Who cares about you on an on-going basis? Do you have a friend who will support you in difficult moments? What, if anything, would stop you from calling a friend in a time of need? If you do not have a close friend you trust to treat you tenderly in times of need, do you have a pet who will listen? *If you do not have a human or animal friend, what do you need to do to get one?* Answer these questions sincerely. Support from others is a critical part of living life well. In fact, I suggest that you give a close friend (*your buddy*) a photocopy of your Progress Plan.

Example: Continuing to Live Life Well

Donna found this book to be helpful. She had recently separated from her husband of 15 years. She lived with their three children and worked forty hours a week. Donna used the book to revise her explanations about her marital separation. As she blamed herself less, she became more interested in knowing herself more deeply. She planned behavioral change programs to help her care for her emotional needs more thoughtfully. Donna began to practice breathing and acceptance exercises in the early morning before her children awakened. She recognized her anger at her situation and began working out with an exercise video to release some of her frustrations. She stopped expressing sheer anger to her husband and worked to state opinions and preferences clearly and responsibly. Donna wanted to strengthen her belief and practice of certain assertive rights. She decided to see a counselor at her health maintenance organization. The counselor supported Donna's plan to apply principles of assertive and creative expression in her new life context.

After going through this chapter, Donna identified several specific skills that were useful to her. She made a commitment to continue to use them. These skills included the following.

1. On-going awareness of how she explained the situations she confronted
2. Breathing and awareness practice in combination with the Daily Caring exercise
3. Application of problem-solving skills
4. Responsible assertive behavior
5. Creative expression activities

Donna identified strong values of self-awareness, intentional action, caring actions toward self and others, responsible behavior, and playfulness. She found that activities demonstrating a value of playfulness were lacking in her lifestyle and decided to attend a stand-up comedy workshop at her church. She planned to review her progress in "being playful" on a weekly basis. Donna also took stock of her social support network. She identified her mother, her sisters, and a neighbor as people who would support her in a time of need. Additionally, Donna noted the value of her dog as a friend who would just "be there." Donna formed "A Behavioral Health Plan to Live a Value-Based Life." Her responses served as an on-going guide for her in creating the lifestyle she wanted. A copy of Donna's "Behavioral Health Plan for Living a Value-Based Life" follows.

Behavioral Health Plan: The Progress Plan

This week's plan will help you develop a lifestyle program for the next six months. Your new skills continue to be vulnerable and you will need to be attentive to your progress. The Progress Plan details your plans concerning monitoring of your progress, practice of coping strategies, lifestyle goals, and emergency plans. Complete it now. The first section concerns **monitoring**. Indicate the method you will use to assess your on-going progress. You may use any of the three methods suggested in this program or a combination of several. Indicate how often you will monitor and when. Be specific. The second section concerns your **plan about using specific coping strategies**. Refer back to your responses to the Review of Strategies Exercise. On your Progress Plan, record the two or three strategies that you rated as most helpful to you at this time in your life. The third section of the Progress Plan refers to **specific lifestyle goals** that you want to set for the next six months. Review your responses to the Values and Lifestyle Exercise and the Behavioral Health Plan to Live a Value-Based Life Exercise. On your Progress Plan, indicate three or four lifestyle goals. These goals may concern maintaining your participation in certain

DONNA'S BEHAVIORAL HEALTH PLAN TO LIVE A VALUE-BASED LIFE	
In living life well, I will:	My Plan
1. Enjoy moments alone by doing things like	**Take a bubble bath by candle light**
2. Set and accomplish goals	**Plan an activity to help me be playful every week**
3. Talk with others in ways that are consistent with my values	**Be assertive in my interactions with the children's father**
4. Create moments of contentment in my work	**Maintain a list of projects I complete**
5. Experience life with my mind *and* body, valuing all of my senses, by engaging in activities I value	**Baking bread, growing flowers and strawberries**
6. Be present and take time to have fun and be playful with others by doing things like	**Spend 30 minutes alone with each of my children every week doing something she/he chooses**
7. Cultivate an attitude of acceptance toward negative feelings and images and know that painful moments, like enchanting experiences, will come and go.	**Caring Moment, breathing work**
I plan to review this commitment:	☐ daily ☒ weekly ☐ monthly
I am 100% committed to this Plan	☒ Yes ☐ No
I will share my plan with: **Doris, my neighbor**	

activities. Additionally, one or two goals may concern exploring new ways to improve your quality of life in areas that continue to be somewhat troubling for you.

The last section of The Progress Plan involves planning for an **emergency**. In this section record how you will know you are in an emergency situation. Link this to your assessment method. For example, if you are using the Quality of Life Scale, you might define an emergency as very low scores for two consecutive weeks. If you are using the Symptoms Checklist, you might define an emergency as endorsing five or more symptoms for two consecutive weeks. Also, indicate your planned response to the emergency. I suggest that you consider the following responses in an emergency situation.

1. Review your Progress Plan.
2. Review important sections of this book.
3. Increase the frequency of engaging in enjoyable, relaxing, pleasurable activities.
4. Plan an outing with a friend.

5. Plan a short vacation to a special area (e.g., the mountains, the ocean, the lake, the forest, a friend's house).

6. Call a friend and discuss problems that are interfering with implementation of your Progress Plan.

7. Call your physician or behavioral health consultant to discuss the emergency and update your Progress Plan.

After you complete your Progress Plan, make several copies. Place one with your bills and one with your important papers. Give one to your buddy. You may want to give a photocopy of your Progress Plan to your health care provider. This may be particularly useful if you are coping with on-going medical problems and have regular contact with a health care team. If you are 100% committed to this plan, you are ready to go forward with your life. You are ready to vitally experience the "ups and downs" of relating to others, working, playing, being in the world and aware of your feelings and choices.

If you have found it hard to follow through with the exercises and strategies presented in this workbook, I recommend that you contact a counselor or other health professional for additional support. Similarly, if your discouragement or depression worsens in spite of sticking with this approach, go for a professional evaluation to see what other treatments might help you. Information on psychotherapy is included in Appendix A. With a little professional support and advice, you will soon be ready to create the lifestyle you want.

References

Beck, A. T., Rush, A. J., Shaw, B. F., & Emery, G. (1979). *Cognitive therapy of depression*. New York, NY: The Guilford Press.

Beck, C. H., & Smith, S. (1993). *Nothing special: Living Zen*. New York, N.Y.: Harper Collins Publishers.

Burns, D. D., & Nolen-Hoeksema, S. (1991). Coping styles, homework compliance, and the effectiveness of cognitive-behavioral therapy. *Journal of Consulting and Clinical Psychology, 59*(2), 305-311.

Ellis, A., & Dryden, W. (1990). *The Essential Albert Ellis*. New York, N.Y.

Kobasa, S. C., & Hilker, R. (1982). Executive work perception and the quality of working life. *Journal of Occupational Medicine, 24*(1), 25-29.

Kobasa, S. C., & Puccetti, M. C. (1983). Personality and social resources in stress resistance. *Journal of Personality and Social Psychology, 45*(4), 839-850.

Kobasa, S. C., Maddi, F. R., & Kahn, F. (1982). Hardiness and health: A prospective study. *Journal of Social Psychology, 42*(1), 168-177.

Kobasa, S. C., Maddi, F. R., & Puccetti, M. C. (1982). Personality and exercises as buffers in the stress-illness relation. *Journal of Behavioral Medicine, 5*(4), 391-404.

Kobasa, S. C., Maddi, F. R., & Zola, M. A. (1983). Type A and hardiness. *Journal of Behavioral Medicine, 6*(1), 41-51.

Kobasa, S. C., Maddi, F. R., Puccetti, M. C. & Zola, M. A. (1985). The effectiveness of hardiness, exercise, and social support as resources against illness. *Journal of Psychosomatic Research, 29*(5), 525-533.

Lewinsohn, P. M., Munoz, R. F., Youngren, M. A., & Zeiss, A. M. (1986). *Control your depression, revised and updated*. New York, NY: Prentice Hall Press.

Marlatt, G. L., & Gordon, J. R. (1985). *Relapse prevention: Maintenance strategies in the treatment of addictive behaviors*. New York, NY: Guilford Press.

Marlatt, G. A., & Tapert, S.F. (1993). Harm reduction: Reducing the risks of addictive behaviors. In J. S. Baer, G. A. Marlatt, & R. J. McMahon (Eds.), *Addictive behaviors across the life span* (pp. 243-273). Newbury Park, CA: Sage Publications.

McClelland, D. C. (1989). Motivational factors in health and disease. Meeting of the American Psychological Association (1988, Atlanta, Georgia). *American Psychologist, 44*(4), 675-683.

McClelland, D. C., Davidson, R. J., & Saron, C. (1985). Stressed power motivation, sympathetic activation, immune function, and illness. *Advances*, Spring, *2*(2), 42-52.

McClelland, D. C., Floor, E., Davidson, R. J., & Saron, C. (1991). Stressed power motivation, sympathetic activation, immune function, and illness. *Journal of Human Stress, 6*(2), 11-19.

Progress Plan

I. Monitoring Plan

To monitor my progress I will use:	☐ The Quality of Life Scale
	☐ The Symptoms Checklist
	☐ The Daily Wellness Check

| I will monitor my progress: | ☐ Weekly   ☐ Every 2 weeks   ☐ Monthly |

| I will monitor my progress on _____ (day of the week). |

II. Specific Coping Strategies

| I plan to use these coping strategies on a daily or weekly basis. |
| 1. |
| 2. |
| 3. |
| 4. |

III. Lifestyle Goals

| I plan to work toward the following lifestyle goals during the next 6 months. |
| 1. |
| 2. |
| 3. |
| 4. |

IV. Emergency Plans

I define an emergency as low scores for 2 weeks on:	☐ The Quality of Life Scale
	☐ The Symptoms Checklist
	☐ The Daily Wellness Check
	☐ Or:

| My emergency plan is to: |
| 1. |
| 2. |
| 3. |
| 4. |

| The person that I am asking to support me in following this plan is: |

Using a Psychologist or Counselor to Help You "Live Life Well"

If your resources for social support are limited and your life problems seem overwhelming, I recommend that you consult a psychologist, counselor, or other health professional. Both counselors and psychologists are specialists in human development and change. They may assist you in developing solutions to life problems and in improving your confidence about your future.

Often, nurses and primary care physicians can provide support to you concerning use of techniques suggested in this book. Nurses and physicians have medical degrees. Psychologists usually have a doctoral degree and counselors usually have a master's degree. All of these professionals are licensed in most states. You can locate a professional by calling your state's referral service lines.

When counseling helps, it is really because of the interaction that occurs between you and the counselor. Finding a helpful psychologist or counselor is sometimes easy and sometimes difficult. Finding a counselor is a little like finding the right apple in a grocery store. Sometimes you put your hand on it first thing. Other times, you need to pass up the first few apples and persevere to find the one that is just right for you. Following is a list of questions to ask yourself after an initial visit to a psychologist or counselor. These questions will help you assess the likelihood of your benefiting from working with that particular professional.

- Did I feel like he or she listened to me?

- Did I feel like he or she understood me?

- Did I feel like we were working together?

- Did I feel like he or she saw me as a capable, creative person that would find solutions to my problems?

- Did I feel like I could disagree with him or her?

Psychologists and counselors are not "above you." They struggle with their own lives and they have specialized training to assist others in improving their lives. Interestingly, over 60% of psychologists responding to a recent survey indicated experience of depression at some point in their lives. You are your best resource for living life well. However, psychologists and counselors may help you apply more effective strategies to problems of living. Sometimes, "two heads are better than one."

References

Pope, K. S., & Tabachnick, B. G. (1994). Therapists as patients: A national survey of psychologists' experiences, problems, and beliefs. Professional Psychology: *Research and Practice, 25*(3), 247-258.

If You Are Considering Using Antidepressant Medications

Medications for depression may be helpful to you. Antidepressant medications relieve troubling symptoms of depression so that you feel more ready to address difficult problems in your life. Your physician will be able to help you make a decision about antidepressant therapy. Consult with your doctor about medication if you are having pronounced difficulties with sleeping, eating, concentration, physical pain, anxiety, and irritability.

If you decide to use medications in your plan to improve the quality of your life, work actively with the person who prescribes these for you. There are a number of different classes of antidepressant medications. Some of these medications have side effects, such as dry mouth and grogginess. Ask your physician about potential side effects and plan specific strategies for coping with anticipated side effects. Report any severe side effects to your doctor. Be attentive to beneficial effects. You will probably notice improvements within the first two weeks of treatment. If you struggle with side effects, your physician may suggest a change to a different class of medication. Most of the time, antidepressant medications are used on a short-term basis–usually 4 to 7 months. Plan the length of antidepressant treatment with your prescribing health care professional and consult with him or her prior to ceasing use of the antidepressant.

The form in Appendix C will help you prepare for a discussion with your health care provider. If you are interested in using medications, complete this form now. Take it with you to your medical appointment.

Medication Information Form*		

Name		Date

History of Medication Use

1. I have taken the following antidepressant in the past:

2. I had the following side effects with this medication:

3. I had the following beneficial effects with this medication:

Current Medications

I am currently using the following medications:

Expectations

I am most troubled by the following problems, which I have marked with an "X." I expect that my treatment, whether I take medications or not, will help with these problems.

1. ☐ Anger or Irritability – often during the day
2. ☐ Sadness – often during the day
3. ☐ Sleep Problems: ☐ too much; ☐ slow to go to sleep; ☐ waking in middle of night; ☐ early morning waking
4. ☐ Interest Problems – a lack of interest in others and in activities I usually enjoy
5. ☐ Guilt, self critical thoughts, feeling inadequate or worthless
6. ☐ Energy Problems – tired most of the time
7. ☐ Concentration Problems
8. ☐ Appetite Change: ☐ significantly greater; ☐ significantly less; ☐ weight loss; ☐ weight gain
9. ☐ Psychomotor Problems: ☐ feeling very "slowed down" or ☐ very "speeded up"
10. ☐ Pain – more aches and more pain
11. ☐ Suicidal thoughts

*Complete and take to your physician if you want to discuss use of antidepressant medications.

Medication Information Form (page 2)*
Beliefs About Use of Medications

I have marked an "X" by statements that I endorse or believe. I am prepared to discuss these with you, as they may influence my successful use of medications.

1. ☐ These kinds of drugs are not the answer to problems in one's life.
1. ☐ These kinds of drugs are a crutch.
1. ☐ I would be the one to get severe side effects.
1. ☐ I should be able to get by without using these kinds of drugs.
1. ☐ I could get addicted.
1. ☐ My family would not want me to use these kinds of drugs.
1. ☐ I will not be able to work if I take these kinds of drugs.
1. ☐ These kinds of drugs are overused.
1. ☐ It is harmful to take too many different kinds of drugs.
1. ☐ These kinds of drugs should not be taken long-term.
1. ☐ Drugs that doctors prescribe for anxiety and depression are dangerous.

*Complete and take to your physician if you want to discuss use of antidepressant medications.

Strategies for Using Medications Successfully

Successful use of medications requires that you follow the following steps:

1. Know the type of medication you are taking and the amount.

2. Know the time of day to take the medication and whether it is best taken with food.

3. Know whether you should make dietary changes while taking the medication.

4. Know the side effects of the medication you are taking and plan ways to cope successfully with these side effects.

5. Develop a collaborative relationship with your prescriber.

6. Know that you should call your prescriber if you are having disturbing symptoms that you attribute to the medication.

7. Monitor beneficial effects.

8. When you are ready to stop using the medication, *plan* discontinuation with your prescriber.

Quality of Life Scale

Emotional Experience

1. Are you experiencing any of the following feelings on a *daily* basis?

☐ Sadness　　☐ Anger　　☐ Fear

2. How intense is your experience of the feelings you checked above? Use this rating scale:

```
1    2    3    4    5    6    7    8    9    10
Not Intense                              Very Intense
```

3. How willing are you to have the feelings you are having? Use this rating scale:

```
1    2    3    4    5    6    7    8    9    10
I cannot tolerate this              I accept this feeling
feeling                             completely
```

Behavioral Action

Using Coping Strategies

During the past week, how often have you used the following coping skills? Use this rating scale:

0 = Not at all　1 = Once　2 = Several times　3 = Almost daily　4 = Daily

1. ___ Participating in pleasurable activities
1. ___ Participating in activities that boost your confidence
1. ___ Simply being aware of an uncomfortable thought, feeling, or emotion without struggling with it
1. ___ Participating in activities that help you relax
1. ___ Using problem-solving techniques for problems you're having in life such as problems with your job or relationships
1. ___ Noticing negative thoughts and replacing them with more realistic thoughts
1. ___ Participating in creative activities

Living Your Values

Please record a number beside each activity to indicate how much you "lived your values" in that area during the past week. Use this rating scale:

```
1    2    3    4    5    6    7    8    9    10
Did Not Live What I                 Lived According to My
Value                               Values
```

1. ___ Enjoying Things Alone　　5. ___ Sensual Experience
1. ___ Accomplishing Things Alone　　1. ___ Fun with Others
1. ___ Talking with Others　　1. ___ Images of a Better Future
1. ___ Contentment with Work

Symptoms Checklist

Please put a check mark by any of the following that have been a problem for you more days than not during the past two weeks.

1. ☐   Anger or Irritability – often during the day

1. ☐   Sadness – often during the day

1. ☐   Sleep Problems: ☐ too much; ☐ slow to go to sleep; ☐ waking in middle of night; ☐ early morning waking

1. ☐   Interest Problems – a lack of interest in others and in activities I usually enjoy

1. ☐   Guilt, self critical thoughts, feeling inadequate or worthless

1. ☐   Energy Problems – tired most of the time

1. ☐   Concentration Problems

1. ☐   Appetite Change: ☐ significantly greater; ☐ significantly less; ☐ weight loss; ☐ weight gain

1. ☐   Psychomotor Problems: ☐ feeling very "slowed down" or ☐ very "speeded up"

1. ☐   More Aches and Pains

1. ☐   Suicidal thoughts

Daily Wellness Check
Date
Rate your quality of life for today. Record positive thoughts or coping strategies associated with the better moments of your life today.

```
     1     2     3     4     5     6     7     8     9    10
  Did not live life well                              Lived life well
```

Thoughts or Activities Related to Rating
1.
2.
3.
4.

Classes That May Help You Develop
Greater Appreciation of Your Mind and Body

- Relaxation Training Workshops
- Breathing Re-Training Classes
- Yoga Classes
- Autogenics Programs
- Body Scan Classes
- Tai Chi Classes
- Sensory Awareness Workshops
- Stretching and Flexibility Classes
- Eurythmy Classes
- Improvisational Theater Programs
- Stand-up Comedy Classes